JN255737

Kyoto Classification of Gastritis

Supervising Editor
Ken Haruma

Editors:
Mototsugu Kato
Kazuhiko Inoue
Kazunari Murakami
Tomoari Kamada

Nihon Medical Center

Kyoto Classification of Gastritis

Supervising Editor   Ken Haruma

Editors   Mototsugu Kato

                                 Kazuhiko Inoue

                                 Kazunari Murakami

                                 Tomoari Kamada

Copyright © 2017 by Nihon Medical Center, Inc.

1-64 Kanda-jinbo-cho, Chiyoda-ku, Tokyo 101-0051, Japan

All rights reserved.

Any reproduction or other unauthorized use of the material or images herein is prohibited without the prior permission of the publisher.

First published in Japanese on September 15, 2014 by Nihon Medical Center, Inc.

English edition published on September 15 , 2017

English Translation   Atsushi Chiba

ISBN: 978-4-88875-298-5

Kyoto Classification of Gastritis

胃炎の京都分類〔英語版〕

2017 年 9 月 15 日　第 1 版 1 刷発行

監　修	春間　賢
編　集	加藤　元嗣, 井上　和彦, 村上　和成, 鎌田　智有
発行者	増永　和也
発行所	株式会社日本メディカルセンター
	東京都千代田区神田神保町 1-64 （神保町協和ビル）
	〒101-0051　TEL 03（3291）3901 ㈹
印刷所	株式会社アイワード

ISBN978-4-88875-298-5

©2017　乱丁・落丁は，お取り替えいたします.

本書に掲載された著作物の複製・転載およびデータベースへの取り込みに関する許諾権は日本メディカルセンターが保有しています.

JCOPY ＜出版者著作権管理機構 委託出版物＞

本書のコピーやスキャン等による無断複製は著作権法上での例外を除き禁じられています. 複製される場合は，そのつど事前に，出版者著作権管理機構（電話 03-3513-6969，FAX03-3513-6979，e-mail：info@jcopy.or.jp）の許諾を得てください.

Preface

In this book, we will present and discuss the endoscopic findings required for diagnosis of gastritis in daily clinical practice with a view to standardize the endoscopic diagnosis of gastritis in Japan.

Initially, the techniques used to diagnose gastritis were developed based on histopathological examinations of autopsied and resected stomachs. Diagnoses of gastritis were based on findings of erosion and inflammation of mucosa, as well as hypertrophy, atrophy, and intestinal metaplasia. Subsequently, the development of gastrocameras and fiberscopes made it possible to observe the gastric mucosa with the naked eye, enabling physicians to diagnose gastritis by looking at optically captured images of actual live tissue. This also made it possible to perform target biopsies; in other words, evaluation of microscopic histopathological images with gastric biopsy was now added to surface observation with endoscopy. The net result of these developments was a huge leap forward in the diagnosis and classification of gastritis.

The primary purpose for diagnosis of gastritis is evaluation of gastric mucosa, as this presents a potential risk of developing gastric cancer. Today, thanks to advances in endoscopic technology, it is now possible to observe gastric mucosa in minute detail. Detection of even minor gastric mucosal changes is now commonplace, leading to a proliferation of endoscopic findings and significantly increasing the complexity of gastritis classification.

However, with the discovery of *Helicobacter pylori* (hereinafter referred to as *H. pylori*) the major cause of gastritis became clear. Taking this discovery into account, the Sydney System was created for classification and grading of gastritis. It was later revised as the Updated Sydney System. Because it incorporates the impact of *H. pylori* infection, this breakthrough system effectively evaluates localization of gastritis and histopathological grading of gastritis, as well as category-specific endoscopic findings and diagnoses.

In Japan, the Kimura-Takemoto Classification of atrophic pattern and the Gastritis Study Group Classification remain the dominant standards in clinical practice. However, in order to bring the Japanese system in line with international practice, introduction of the Updated Sydney System was inevitable as it is the common available standard. Regardless, Japan already has a well-established and long-standing historical background in gastritis classification. It also happens to have a high occurrence of gastric cancer. What Japan needs now is a gastric diagnosis system that evaluates the risk of gastric cancer.

From the 10th to 12th of May, 2013, I presided over the 85th Congress of the Japan Gastroenterological Endoscopy Society at the Kyoto International Conference Center. Two main themes in gastritis diagnosis were discussed at this meeting. One was how to clarify the findings used to diagnose *H. pylori*-infected gastritis in standard endoscopic diagnostics in Japan while striving for greater objectivity and higher accuracy in endoscopic findings, as well as in histopathological findings based on the Updated Sydney System. The other topic was to develop a method for grading gastritis that could evaluate a risk of gastric cancer.

This book features images and accompanying descriptions that can be used as a basis for diagnosis of gastritis. The physicians who contributed to this book include many who participated in the discussions at the 85th Congress, as well as others who are engaged in everyday practice of gastritis diagnosis. During the preparation of this book, we held dozens of face-to-face meetings and communicated constantly via the Internet to ensure that we were all agreed on the classifications described herein.

As both supervising editor and contributing author, I look forward to seeing this classification system validated in clinical cases, and hope that it will be upgraded regularly, and evaluated internationally.

May 2017

Ken Haruma
Professor, General Internal Medicine 2,
General Medical Center,
Kawasaki Medical School

■ Supervising Editor

Ken Haruma — Professor, General Internal Medicine 2, General Medical Center, Kawasaki Medical School

■ Editors

Mototsugu Kato — Director, National Hospital Organization Hakodate Hospital

Kazuhiko Inoue — Associate Professor, Department of General Medicine, Kawasaki Medical School

Kazunari Murakami — Professor, Faculty of Medicine, Oita University

Tomoari Kamada — Professor, Department of Health Care Medicine, Kawasaki Medical School

■ Authors: (in order of appearance)

Ken Haruma — Professor, General Internal Medicine 2, General Medical Center, Kawasaki Medical School

Tomoari Kamada — Professor, Department of Health Care Medicine, Kawasaki Medical School

Kazunari Murakami — Professor, Faculty of Medicine, Oita University

Masashi Kawamura — Chief Physician, Department of Gastroenterology, Sendai City Hospital

Shuichi Terao — Vice Hospital President/Supervising Director of Department of Gastroenterology, Kakogawa Central Hospital

Takahiro Kato — Professor, Department of Gastroenterology, Murakami Memorial Hospital, Asahi University

Yutaka Yamaji — Department of Gastroenterology, University of Tokyo

Yoshihiro Hirata — Specially Appointed Lecturer, Department of Gastroenterology, University of Tokyo

Masanori Ito — Associate Professor, Department of Gastroenterology and Metabolism, Hiroshima University

Shinji Kitamura — Assistant Professor, Department of Gastroenterology and Oncology, Tokushima University School of Biomedical Sciences

Kazuyoshi Yagi — Professor, Department of Gastroenterology and Hepatology, Uonuma Institute of Community Medicine, Niigata University Medical and Dental Hospital

Kazuhiko Inoue — Associate Professor, Department of General Medicine, Kawasaki Medical School

Susumu Ohwada — Inui Clinic of Internal Medicine; Director, Gastroenterology and Oncology Center, IMS Ohta Chuo General Hospital

Masayuki Inui — President, Inui Clinic of Internal Medicine

Naondo Sohara — Vice President, Shirakawa Clinic

Yoshikatsu Inui — Vice President, Inui Clinic of Internal Medicine

Takashi Kawai — Professor, Gastroenterological Endoscopy, Tokyo Medical University

Hironori Masuyama — President, Masuyama Gastrointestinal Clinic

Shigemi Nakajima — Director, Department of General Medicine, Japan Community Healthcare Organization (JCHO) Shiga Hospital

Mitsugi Yasuda — Director, Ningen Dock Center, KKR Takamatsu Hospital

Mototsugu Kato — Director, National Hospital Organization Hakodate Hospital

Katsuhiro Mabe — Contact Assistant Professor, Department of Cancer Preventive Medicine, Hokkaido University Graduate School of Medicine

Ryoji Kushima — Professor, Division of Diagnostic Pathology, Shiga University of Medical Science

Contents

Kyoto Classification of Gastritis

Chapter 1 History of the Classification of Gastritis
Ken Haruma　7

① History of Gastritis Classification / 12

② Purpose of the Kyoto Classification /18

Chapter 2 Endoscopic Findings of Gastritis　　23

1. Introduction　　　　　　　　　　　　　　Tomoari Kamada　25

　① *H. pylori*-uninfected gastric mucosa = Normal stomach / 25

　② Currently *H. pylori*-infected gastric mucosa = Chronic active gastritis (CAG) /26

　③ Previously *H. pylori*-infected gastric mucosa

　　(natural disappearance of *H. pylori* after eradication or advanced atrophy)

　　= Chronic inactive gastritis (CIG) /28

　④ Changes in the gastric mucosa caused by drugs /29

2. Specific Discussions

① Atrophy	Kazunari Murakami	30
② Intestinal metaplasia	Masashi Kawamura	33
③ Diffuse redness	Shuichi Terao	38
④ Spotty redness	Shuichi Terao	43
⑤ Mucosal swelling	Takahiro Kato	46
⑥ Enlarged folds and tortuous folds	Yutaka Yamaji, Yoshihiro Hirata	49
⑦ Nodularity	Tomoari Kamada	52
⑧ Foveolar-hyperplastic polyp	Masanori Ito	57
⑨ Xanthoma	Shinji Kitamura	60
⑩ Depressive erosion	Yoshihiro Hirata	63
⑪ Regular arrangement of collecting venules (RAC)	Kazuyoshi Yagi	66
⑫ Fundic gland polyp	Kazuhiko Inoue	68
⑬ Red streak	Susumu Ohwada, et al.	71
⑭ Raised erosion	Takashi Kawai	75
⑮ Hematin	Hironori Masuyama	77
⑯ Corpus erosion	Shigemi Nakajima	79
⑰ Patchy redness	Masashi Kawamura	83
⑱ Map-like redness	Mitsugi Yasuda	88
⑲ Multiple white and flat elevated lesions	Tomoari Kamada	91
Additional Information: Cobblestone Mucosa	Tomoari Kamada	94

Chapter 3 Endoscopic Findings for Risk Stratification of Gastric Cancer   97

1. Description   Mototsugu Kato   99

　① Relationship between gastric cancer and background gastritis / 99

　② Endoscopic findings related to the risk of gastric cancer / 101

　③ Scores for endoscopic findings related to the risk of gastric cancer / 101

2. Clinical Cases   Tomoari Kamada   104

Chapter 4 Recording Endoscopic Findings of Gastritis
                                                                        111

1. Description and Clinical Cases   Katsuhiro Mabe   113

　① Basic method for entering data / 113

　② Entering endoscopic findings of gastritis according to clinical cases / 114

2. Check Sheet for Background Gastric Mucosa in Endoscopy

　　　— Also usable for checkups for gastric cancer and other gastrointestinal diseases
                                                   Kazuhiko Inoue, et al.   118

3. Endoscopic Diagnosis and Classification of Chronic Gastritis

　　　That Conforms to Histological Diagnosis   Shigemi Nakajima, et al. 121

　① Diagnosis policy of chronic gastritis / 121

　② Diagnosis of presence/absence and activity of chronic gastritis / 121

　③ Diagnosis of atrophy / 123

　④ Consistency with pathological diagnosis / 123

Cover photos courtesy of Division of Gastroenterology, Kawasaki Medical School

Chapter 1

History of the Classification of Gastritis

Chapter 1　History of the Classification of Gastritis

Ken Haruma

Introduction — Background of the Classification of Gastritis

Gastritis is classified into acute gastritis and chronic gastritis according to the clinical course. When the term of gastritis is used, however, it usually refers to chronic gastritis. The onset of acute gastritis is characterized by sudden epigastric pain, nausea, and vomiting — particularly hematemesis and melena. In daily clinical practice, it is often diagnosed based on the patient's medical history and physical examination findings. Characteristic findings of acute gastritis include indications of multiple erosions and shallow ulcers with blood coagulation in upper gastrointestinal endoscopy. These are also called acute gastric mucosal lesions (AGMLs).

In daily practice in Japan, the term chronic gastritis has three different usages. The first is in diagnosis and treatment where it is used when patients complain of symptoms such as epigastric pain, upset stomach, and nausea (symptomatic gastritis). The second is when morphologic abnormalities are recognized in endoscopy and X-ray examination (morphological gastritis). And the third is in histopathological diagnosis in which gastric biopsy specimens are collected (histological gastritis).

However, morphological gastritis and histological gastritis are not necessarily accompanied by subjective symptoms, while many cases of histological gastritis are now known to be caused by *Helicobacter pylori* (hereinafter referred to as *H. pylori*) infection. Haphazard use of the term "chronic gastritis" has led to insistence that it only be used only when a definitive diagnosis is made histopathologically — which is the way how it should have been in the first place. Now, cases presenting gastrointestinal symptoms centering around the epigastric region are diagnosed as functional dyspepsia (FD), although organic disorders such as peptic ulcer and gastric cancer that can be the cause of the symptoms are not recognized. As far as insurance-covered diagnosis and treatment, this is also the case in Japan. Since the discovery of *H. pylori*, morphological gastritis diagnosed endoscopically is now seen as the precursor of gastric cancer and peptic ulcers, as well as an index for easy screening of *H. pylori* infection.

Diagnosis of gastritis began with histopathological diagnosis of autopsied and resected stomachs. Subsequent advances in the study of subjective symptoms led to further clinical progress. When gastrocameras and fiberscopes arrived on the scene, physicians were able to diagnose gastritis using findings obtained from direct observation of the gastric mucosa. As soon as it was possible to collect biopsied gastric tissue, histopathological diagnosis of gastritis became an active field of study. For example, Konjetzny's histopathological study using resected stomachs[2] and Schindler's study on diagnosis and classification of gastritis using a flexible gastrocamera[1, 6, 9, 28] significantly contributed to subsequent advancement in diagnosis of gastritis using endoscopes (**Fig. 1**). Later, Schindler's diagnostics of gastritis was

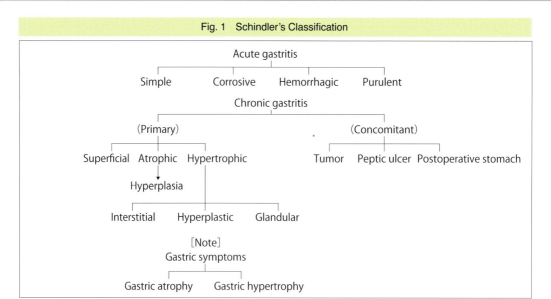

Fig. 1 Schindler's Classification

revalidated and studied in detail by our great predecessors in Japan[3)-5), 7)-19), 21)-27), 29)-31), 33), 34), 36)-41), 43), 44)], who added Japanese-original diagnostics to the methodology. Today, the resulting diagnostic system continues to be used in daily practice[49-52), 59), 60), 63)-65), 69), 71), 76), 83)-85)].

Schindler's work played a crucial role in increasing the effectiveness of diagnosis of gastritis and in the years following the mortality rate of gastric cancer significantly declined in Europe and North America. Today, endoscopic diagnosis and classification of gastritis is rarely performed except in those countries where the mortality rate of gastric cancer is still high. One of those countries is Japan. Not surprisingly, with such a high incidence of gastric cancer, the study of gastritis — which is a precursor for gastric cancer — is flourishing in Japan.

Due to advances in imaging diagnosis which have made possible early detection of gastric cancer using gastric X-ray examinations and endoscopy, changes in gastric mucosa such as atrophy and intestinal metaplasia can now be detected and used as findings to differentiate gastric cancer. Detailed classification of these findings has led to the creation of the Kimura-Takemoto Classification system [27), 31)] **(Fig. 2)**. This leading-edge Japanese study is now used in daily practice.

In 1983, Warren and Marshall discovered *H. pylori*[45)]. The establishment of *H. pylori* as a leading cause of histological gastritis precipitated a monumental revolution in gastritis diagnostics. Determining the presence or absence of *H. pylori* infection in endoscopic findings is a key element in diagnosis, making it more necessary than ever to precisely diagnose whether gastritis is a high risk for gastric cancer.

Against this background, the Sydney System was proposed[55)] as internationally standardized diagnostic criteria by a group of researchers from six countries in Europe and North America at the 9th World Congress of Gastroenterology held in Sydney in 1990. As data on causes, localization, histopathological images, and endoscopic findings of gastritis continued to accumulate in the years that followed, the Sydney System for the classification and grading of gastritis was revised in 1996 in what became known as the Updated Sydney System[68)] **(Fig. 3)**. As well as taking the presence or absence of *H. pylori* infection into consideration, this system

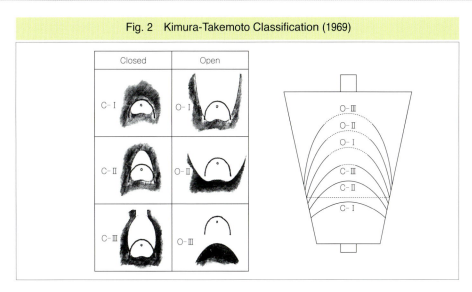

Fig. 2 Kimura-Takemoto Classification (1969)

[Kimura K, et al. Excerpted from Endoscopy. 1969; 1 (3): 87-96[27].]
Note: Although the degrees of atrophy are graded as C-1, C-2, C-3, O-1, O-2, and O-3 in this book, the grading system in the original article is used in this figure.

explained endoscopic findings, analyzed assessments of endoscopic gastritis, and classified histopathological findings into four grades. The comprehensiveness and reliability of the Updated Sydney System led it to becoming the standard in Japan as well.

Nevertheless, there are some problems with the Sydney System; for one, an objective diagnosis is difficult with some of the endoscopic findings discussed. Other problems for us in Japan include the fact that there is no mention of the Kimura-Takemoto Classification[27], which is commonly used for evaluation of progress of atrophic gastritis in Japan, nor of nodular gastritis[81], which can cause a high risk of undifferentiated cancer.

At the 85th Congress of the Japan Gastroenterological Endoscopy Society held in Kyoto in May 2013, two main themes in gastritis diagnosis were discussed with an eye to resolving the problems with the Updated Sydney System. One was how to clarify the findings used to diagnose *H. pylori*-infected gastritis in standard endoscopic diagnostics in Japan while striving for greater objectivity and higher accuracy in endoscopic findings, as well as in histopathological findings based on the Updated Sydney System. The other topic was to develop a method for grading gastritis that could pose a risk of gastric cancer. While taking into account the diagnostics and classification of gastritis already developed in Japan, as well as building on the foundation of diagnosis of *H. pylori* infection and evaluation of gastric cancer risks, we clarified gastritis findings in a manner we considered objective, convenient, and clinically significant. After repeated meetings and back-and-forth over the Internet between those of us who made presentations at the congress and many other endoscopists active in clinical practice in various fields, the classification system was finalized. The result is the proposed "Kyoto Classification of Gastritis."

This chapter outlines diagnosis and classification of gastritis around the world up until the present and summarizes the historical background that has led to the Kyoto Classification. To make it easier to understand the historical transition, references are listed in chronological order.

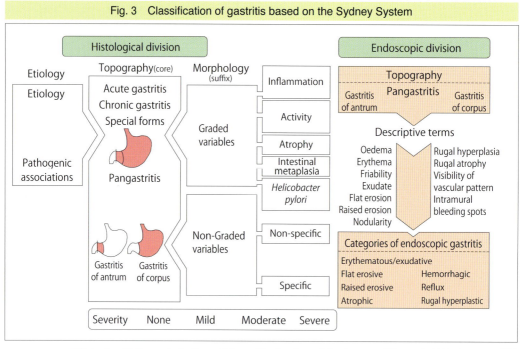

[Misiewicz JJ. Excerpted with partial modification from J Gastroenterol Hepatol. 1991: 6: 207-208[57].]

History of Gastritis Classification

When we look back at the history of the classification of gastritis, we find a wide array of papers and books written by our illustrious predecessors based on detailed studies of earlier material. Having looked at as much of this material as I could get my hands on, I have put together a history of gastritis classification based on the literature and my own thoughts on the subject.

1) Schindler's classification and classifications based on it

According to the paper by Ichioka[21], the existence of gastritis had already been established in the 18th century and continued to be further clarified according to anatomical findings up to the beginning of the 19th century. In 1922, Schindler was the first to point out the existence of endoscopic gastritis by observing the gastric mucosa with a gastroscope.

Then in 1932, Schindler and Wolf created a flexible gastroscope that was easy to insert and contributed to gradual clarification of endoscopic images of chronic gastritis[1,9]. 1n 1947, Schindler published his landmark work Gastrits[9], which included some modifications to Konjetzny's histopathological studies[2] using resected stomachs. Schindler divided chronic gastritis into primary gastritis and concomitant gastritis accompanied by gastric cancer and peptic ulcer. He also classified primary gastritis into three types: chronic superficial gastritis, chronic atrophic gastritis, and chronic hypertrophic gastritis[6,9] (Fig. 1).

Meanwhile in Japan in 1936, Tagawa, who was already using the term "erosive gastritis", classified chronic gastritis into three types: superficial gastritis, hypertrophic gastritis, and atrophic gastritis[3].

From the 1940s to the 1960s, many pioneering researchers in Japan conducted extensive studies of the stomach, eventually established original detailed diagnostics for chronic gastritis based on Schindler's endoscopic classification. It was against this background that gastritis

Table 1 Tasaka's Classification (1956)	Table 2 Sakita's Classification

I. Primary gastritis
  1. Superficial gastritis
  2. Atrophic gastritis
    a. Atrophic
    b. Superficial atrophic
    c. Atrophic hyperplastic
  3. Hypertrophic gastritis
II. Concomitant gastritis
	1. Superficial gastritis
	2. Hypertrophic gastritis
	  1) Proliferative hypertrophic gastritis
	  2) Interstitial hypertrophic gastritis
	  3) Glandular hypertrophic gastritis
	3. Atrophic gastritis
	  1) Atrophic (simple) gastritis
	  2) Superficial atrophic gastritis
	  3) Atrophic hyperplastic gastritis
	  4) Atrophic intestinal metaplastic gastritis
	  5) Atrophic hyperplastic intestinal metaplastic gastritis

[Tasaka S, et al. Excerpted from Sogo Rinsho.1956; 5: 1–9[10].]

[Sakita T. Excerpted from Gendai Iryo. 1982; 14: 227[46].]

classifications of Tasaka, Sakita, Yamagata, et al. were created **(Tables 1–3)**.

While the classifications were being established, many clinical studies were conducted. These included studies of histopathological images of hyperplastic gastritis and clinical courses of chronic gastritis, as well as histopathological images of concomitant gastritis and other functional changes such as gastric acid secretion[46].

Today, modern videoscopes make it easy to observe gastric mucosa in detail thanks to their slim insertion tubes, easy handling, and powerful imaging capability. When you look at what our predecessors were able to achieve using the gastroscopes and clumsy, old-fashioned fiberscopes that were available at the time, it is all the more impressive.

2) Kimura-Takemoto Classification

When fiberscopes that made possible endoscopic biopsies were developed, diagnosis of gastritis took a huge leap forward — atrophic gastritis in particular. Kimura and Takemoto compared biopsied gastric tissues with fiberscopic findings to establish diagnostic criteria for atrophic gastritis. He later determined that the glandular border between the pyloric and fundic glands appeared at the lesser curvature of the angulus and defined it as an endoscopic atrophic border in 1966. It was later clarified that the border extended to the proximal side when the atrophy in the corpus progressed. In 1969, this was introduced as the Kimura-Takemoto Classification[27] (Fig. 2). Because it simplified endoscopic evaluation of the degree of atrophy in the corpus, the Kiumra-Takekmoto Classification soon became a key part of diagnosis and grading of gastritis in Japan. However, having personally had the opportunity to participate in or observe endoscopies in Germany, Britain, the United States, Brazil, Chile, India, Cambodia, and China, I have noticed that clinical cases in which an atrophic band was found in the lesser curvature of the angulus are extremely rare, except in Chile. For this reason, the Kiumra-Takekmoto Classification was not incorporated into the Sydney System, despite the fact that it makes possible easy, accurate diagnosis of the degree of atrophic gastritis and has been used in Japan for everyday diagnosis of gastritis for more than four decades.

3) Classification of the Study Group for Establishing Endoscopic Diagnosis of Chronic Gastritis

In the 1990s, the Study Group for Establishing Endoscopic Diagnosis of Chronic Gastritis was founded, and the group's first classification was presented at the 10th Meeting for Gastritis Study which was held on October 19, 1995 **(Table 4)**. The basic purpose of this tentative

Chapter 1 History of the Classification of Gastritis

Table 3　Yamagata's Classification

Endoscopic findings

1. Superficial gastritis
   a. Attachment of mucus
      When grayish white mucus is attached diffusely or in patches
   b. Patchy redness
      When the mucosa is reddish with unclear boundaries caused by partial expansion
      and contraction of superficial capillaries
   c. Edema
      When the mucosa grows pale, swells, or becomes very glossy
2. Atrophic gastritis
   1) Simple atrophic change
      a. Mucosal discoloration: Gray, grayish green, grayish yellow
      b. Visible vascular pattern
      c. Bright image
   2) Superficial gastritis change
      When the above superficial changes and erosion are present concurrently
   3) Hyperplastic change
      When stiff verrucous mucosa and nodular mucosal elevation are exhibited and
      vascular pattern becomes indistinct
   4) Intestinal metaplastic change
      Peculiar patchy mucosal discoloration
3. Hypertrophic gastritis
   Soft elevation of mucosal surface

[Yamagata S, et. al. Excerpted from Iji Shinpo. 1961; 1916: 5–16[15].]

classification was to coordinate and generalize the various gastritis classifications proposed up to that point, as well as to create a new classification system that would be useful in everyday endoscopy. The guiding principles included: ① it should be simple; ② it should extend conventional classifications — meaning that it would incorporate Schindler's, Tasaka's, and Sakita's classifications as its basis, while including Sano's clinical histopathological classification[44]; ③ it should serve as a practical endoscopic classification backed up by histopathological findings; ④ it should grade locality, severity, and activity and assign those grades to the names of diseases, as well as identify causes and autoimmune mechanisms where possible; and ⑤ and, finally, it should take into account the Sydney System. The utility of this tentative gastritis classification was confirmed in a comparison with histological gastritis and diagnosis of *H. pylori* infection.

4) Discovery of *H. pylori* and proposal of the Sydney System

In 1983, Warren, Marshall, et al. discovered *H. pylori* in the gastric mucosa of gastritis patients[45]. This discovery shattered the existing understanding of gastritis, revolutionizing diagnosis of gastritis. In other words, it made it essential to take into account mucosal damage wrought by cytokines and chemical substances generated from inflammatory cells such as polymorphonuclear cells and mononuclear cells that are induced to the gastric mucosa. It also made it clear that external factors played a less significant role in gastritis than had been previously thought.Against this background, the Sydney System[55), 68)] was proposed in 1990 by European gastroenterologists and pathologists in order to standardize the classification of

| Table 4 | Classification of the Study Group for Establishing Endoscopic Diagnosis of Chronic Gastritis (revised tentative draft) (1995) |

I. Basic types
  (1) Superficial gastritis
  (2) Hemorrhagic gastritis
  (3) Erosive gastritis
  (4) Atrophic gastritis
  (5) Verrucous gastritis
  (6) Metaplastic gastritis
  (7) Hyperplastic gastritis
II. Mixed types
  Superficial atrophic gastritis
  Atrophic hyperplastic gastritis
  Other
III. Special types

[10th Meeting for Gastritis Study. Excerpted from Ther Res. 1995; 16: 37–41[67].]

gastritis. The Sydney System (Fig. 3) stipulated the world's common diagnostic criteria, compiling all the causes, locality, histopathological images, and endoscopic findings available at the time. This classification emphasized the importance of *H. pylori* infection as the cause of gastritis. The locality of gastritis was classified into antral gastritis, corpus gastritis, and pangastritis. In addition, a grading system was developed in which histopathological findings were classified into chronic inflammation, neutrophil activity, atrophy, and intestinal metaplasia, while the amount of *H. pylori* bacteria was specified as none, mild, moderate, or severe. Eleven different endoscopic findings were incorporated in this classification system, including edema, erythema, friability, exudate, and erosion. However, there were a number of problems with the system. These included difficulty in objectively evaluating findings such as friability and exudate, intermingling of endoscopic findings and pathological findings, and the fact that nodular change was listed as an endoscopic finding, despite there being no corresponding endoscopic classification.

According to the Sydney System, findings that would suggest *H. pylori* infection included diffuse erythema, spotty erythema, edema, and mucus attachment. However, these findings had already been classified as superficial by Schindler, when he first established the diagnostics of gastritis using a gastroscope in the 1920s. In Schindler's classification, superficial gastritis included "red patches, layers of adherent, glary, grayish mucus." His original book reported that the histological findings in the pyloric gland region showed localized presence of inflammatory cell infiltration in the foveolar epithelial region in the upper half of the mucosa. As far as I am concerned, this is nothing but superficial gastritis. When he performed follow-up observation of superficial gastritis, Schindler reported that about half had returned to normal, while the remainder had advanced to atrophy. Cases of acute *H. pylori* infection tend to either disappear on their own and go into remission or continue and progress to atrophy. Schindler's report seems to precisely reflect this transition. When atrophy progresses in the gastric corpus and viscous mucus is attached, this is obviously a finding that shows mucus attachment. However, the findings of mucus attachment found in the antrum of the stomach shown in the original version of the Sydney System are pretty difficult to diagnose when the mucus is treated prior to endoscopy.

The term "erosive gastritis," first appeared in the Gutzeit-Teitge Classification or Boller Classification presented in 1954. According to Sada's paper[36], Palmer further subclassified erosive gastritis into acute erosion and chronic erosion. Subsequently, Walk subclassified it into a type with either very slight or no elevation at all around the erosion (punctiform) and a type with noticeable elevation on the surrounding mucosa (varioliform).

Further studies of erosive gastritis using endoscopic findings and resected stomachs were subsequently carried out in Japan. Since the discovery of *H. pylori*, it has been understood that raised erosive gastritis in the antrum is usually *H. pylori* negative. Erosive redness, on the other hand, is widely regarded as a specific finding indicating *H. pylori*-caused gastritis. In daily practice, this is a finding worthy of attention, as is atrophy in the corpus according to the Kimura-Takemoto Classification, RAC, and alteration in the folds of the corpus. Edema also appears in the Updated Sydney System and is another specific finding for *H. pylori*-infected gastritis. It has been pointed out that erosive redness is also a finding in portal hypertension[47), 53), 65)] accompanied by hepatic cirrhosis. In this case, a clear image diagnosis is required.

5) Histopathological classification of gastritis

Initially, diagnosis and classification of gastritis was based on histopathological examinations using autopsied and resected stomachs. Later, as it became possible to collect biopsied stomach tissue, and with subsequent advances in endoscopic technology making it easier to biopsy tissues endoscopically, more refined classification systems were developed using biopsied stomach tissue[20), 31), 32), 48)]. When Whitehead et al. attempted to classify gastritis histopathologically in 1972, they proposed clear definitions of pyloric gland mucosa and fundic gland mucosa. They also described different degrees of gastritis, noted the presence/absence and degree of intestinal metaplasia, and evaluated the different degrees of neutrophil infiltration[32]. Today, these guidelines are widely used by pathologists for histopathological classification, just as Schindler's guidelines are used in clinical classification. In Whitehead's Classification, inflammatory cell infiltration near the superficial layer of the mucosa is regarded as superficial gastritis without considering the presence or absence of atrophy. Guidelines published later classified cases without atrophy of fundic glands — although inflammatory cellular infiltration is recognized — as superficial gastritis. As we have seen, the same superficial gastritis can be interpreted in different ways depending on the classification system used. In Japan, well-known publications by pathologists such as Yoshii and Sano[43), 44)], as well as Hirafuku's histological classification[26] have proven convenient and easy to use **(Fig. 4)**. I have used these works as references in all my past studies[42), 56), 58), 61), 66), 70), 72)–75), 77)]. Today, the Updated Sydney System's grading system, which is categorized into inflammation, activity, atrophy, and intestinal metaplasia, is widely used. More recently, Rugge et al. built on the Sydney System to create a histological risk classification for gastric cancer[78), 79), 82)].

6) Classification of autoimmune gastritis

In 1973, Strickland and Mackay described functional aspects of autoimmune gastritis such as gastric acid secretion and blood gastrin in addition to morphology[35] **(Table. 5)**. Autoimmune gastritis is especially prevalent in North America and Europe, particularly in the Scandinavian region. Strickland and Mackay's prime focus was on autoimmunity as a generating factor of chronic gastritis and local anatomic sites of inflammation. They classified this type of gastritis into Type A and Type B.

Type A gastritis was distinguished by hypergastrinemia and positive antiparietal cell antibodies with atrophic changes mainly in the fundic gland region. Its onset was considered to be

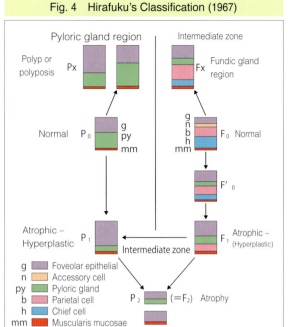

Fig. 4 Hirafuku's Classification (1967)

[Hirafuku I. Excerpted from I to Cho (Stomach Intest), 1967; 2: 1257–1264[26].]

Table 5 Classification of chronic gastritis by Strickland & Mackay (1973)

	Type A gastritis	Type B gastritis
Atrophic region	Mainly in cardia/corpus (Fundic gland region)	Mainly in pyloric region (Pyloric gland region)
Antral inflammation	±	+++
Acid secretion	↓↓↓	↓
Anti-parietal cell antibody	+++	—
Anti-intrinsic factor antibody	+	—
Corpus gastritis	+++	+
Serum gastrin level	↑	Normal
Pernicious anemia	With complication	Without complication

[Strickland RG, Mackay IR. Excerpted with modification from Am J Dig Dis, 1973; 18: 426–440[35].]

triggered by an autoimmune mechanism that created antibodies that attacked the parietal cells. It was typically observed in the stomach with pernicious anemia, and often accompanied by complications such as carcinoid tumors or gastric cancer. Type B gastritis was defined as normal atrophic gastritis with atrophic changes showing mainly in the pyloric gland region with negative antiparietal cell antibodies and hypoacidity. Type B gastritis, which soon came to be referred to as antral gastritis in daily practice, was highly prevalent in Europe and North America. Today, the term Type B gastritis is used for gastritis with hyperacidity.

Table 6 Chronology of major gastritis classifications

1930s	Gastritis classification by Schindler	Bull NY Acad Med, 1939; 15: 322–337[6]
1936	Chronic gastritis classification by Tagawa	J Gastroenterol, 1936; 35: 243–296[3]
1956	Gastritis classification by Tasaka	Sogo Rinsho, 1956; 5: 1–9[10]
1963	Gastritis classification by Yamagata	Iji Shinpo, 1961; 1916: 5–16[15]
1967	Gastritis classification by Hirafuku	I to Cho (Stomach Intest), 1967: 2: 1257–1264[26]
1969	Kimura-Takemoto Classification	Endoscopy, 1969: 1 (3): 87–97[27]
1973	Chronic gastritis classification by Strickland et al.	Am J Dig Dis, 1973: 18: 426–440[35]
1990	Sydney System: Classification and Grading of Gastritis as the Basis of Diagnosis and Treatment	J Gastroenterol Hepatol, 1991; 6: 223–234[55]
1995	Classification of the Study Group for Establishing Endoscopic Diagnosis of Chronic Gastritis	Ther Res, 1995; 16: 37–41[67]
1996	Updated Sydney System: Classification and Grading of Gastritis as the Basis of Diagnosis and Treatment	Am J Surg Pathol, 1996: 20: 1161–1181[68]
2014	Kyoto Classification of Gastritis	This book

Purpose of the Kyoto Classification

Today, endoscopy is used in the diagnosis of gastritis to determine the presence/absence of *H. pylori* infection, as well as to evaluate the risks of gastric cancer and clarify subsequent measures. In the decades since Schindler's use of gastroscopy to establish comprehensive gastritis diagnostic, many studies have been conducted in Japan and elsewhere in the world and new endoscopic findings have been discussed. Yet problems still remain. Papers continue to be produced by well-known doctors[54, 57, 62, 79, 80] — who had been struggling to define gastritis even before the discovery of *H. pylori* — that discuss problems of diagnosis and classification following the discovery of *H. pylori*, as well as the difficulty of clarifying endoscopic findings objectively so that their meaning would be clear to everyone. Our goal is to resolve these issues by carefully reviewing gastritis classification systems developed both here in Japan and around the world, and building on those systems to create a new classification system supplemented by images and corresponding descriptions on a morphological scale that would facilitate objective diagnosis of gastritis findings. At the 85th Congress of the Japan Gastroenterological Endoscopy Society, we focused our discussion on two major areas, following up with numerous conferences with participants that included chairpersons, presenters, and doctors from various fields who were engaged in endoscopy. As well as face-to-face meetings, contributors engaged in dialog via the Internet in an effort to determine which findings and endoscopic images should be included and their endoscopic images, as well as how to establish a reliable method for evaluating the risk of gastric cancer. The results of these efforts came to fruition in this book — Kyoto Classification of Gastritis — which was written by the doctors who took part in the creation of this classification.

Our intent in this book is to present typical images of findings of gastritis to facilitate objective diagnosis, while also taking into account the various gastritis diagnosis and classification systems thus far established. Beyond that, we have attempted to systemize evaluation of risks for gastric cancer. We also take into consideration the previously inconceivable changes that occur in the gastric mucosa after *H. pylori* eradication[77), 84]. Changes in the gastric mucosa caused by drugs such as proton pump inhibitors, antiplatelet agents, and anticoagulant agents are also increasing in frequency, as are changes due to underlying conditions such as renal failure. These too we discuss in this book.

Conclusion

The history of diagnosis and classification in Japan and around the world is outlined in **Table 6**. Schindler's diagnostics of gastritis remains to the foundation for the classification of gastritis even to this day. With its effective classification of atrophic gastritis, the Kimura-Takemoto Classification also remains an invaluable tool and resource. As medical knowledge has progressed, the purpose of gastritis diagnosis has changed. At its core, however, the primary purpose for the diagnosis of gastric mucosa is to determine whether or not there is a risk of gastric cancer. Since the discovery that *H. pylori* was a leading cause of gastritis and peptic ulcers, more attention has been focused on diagnosis of *H. pylori* than on diagnosis of gastritis. However, morphology of the gastric mucosa will continue to change as *H. pylori* infection rates decrease. Changes in the social environment such as evolving eating habits may also impact the nature of gastritis.

I hope that the Kyoto Classification will prove of interest not only to specialists in gastritis, but also to physicians who are active in daily practice and that it will be helpful in clinical practice.

References••••

1) Schindler R. Die diagnostische Bedeutung der Gastroskopie. Mun Med Wochenschr. 1922; 69: 535–537.

2) Konjetzny GE. Entzündungen des Magens. Henke-Lubarsch Handbuch der speziellen pathologischen Anatomie und Histologie (4th Ed). Berlin: Springer-Verlag, 1928.

3) Tagawa J. [Chronic gastritis.] Nippon Shokakibyo Gakkai Zasshi. 1936; 35: 243–296. (In Japanese.)

4) Okada S. [About chronic gastritis (1).] Shokakibyogaku. 1937; 2: 1–12. (In Japanese.)

5) Okada S. [About chronic gastritis (2).] Shokakibyogaku. 1937; 2: 187–209. (In Japanese.)

6) Schindler R. Chronic gastritis. Bull N Y Acad Med, 1939; 15: 322–337.

7) Okinaka S, Kondo D, Kishimoto K. [About gastritis found in gastric and duodenal ulcer patients.] Nippon Shokakibyo Gakkai Zasshi. 1941; 40: 241–243. (In Japanese.)

8) Okinaka S, Kondo D, Kishimoto K. [Gastroscopic study of gastritis: second report on gastritis found in gastric ulcer patients.] Nippon Shokakibyo Gakkai Zasshi. 1943; 42: 301–303.(In Japanese.)

9) Schindler R. Gastritis. New York: Grune & Stratton, 1947.

10) Tasaka S, Takahashi T, Sakita T, et al. [Study of gastric disease using a gastrocamera: first report on chronic gastritis.] Sogo Rinsho. 1956; 5: 1–9. (In Japanese.)

11) Utsumi Y. [Study about chronic gastritis: clinical study mainly using a gastrocamera.] Nippon Shokakibyo Gakkai Zasshi. 1958; 55: 103–131. (In Japanese.)

12) Kasugai T. [Study about gastric disease using a gastrocamera.] Nippon Shokakibyo Gakkai Zasshi. 1959; 56: 637–661. (In Japanese.)

13) Niwa H. [Study about chronic gastritis: follow-up study mainly using a gastrocamera.] Nippon Ikamera Gakkai Kikanshi 1959; 1: 9–29. (In Japanese.)

14) Yamagata S. [Study about endoscopic diagnostics.] Nippon Shokakibyo Gakkai Zasshi. 1961; 58: 645–

654. (In Japanese.)

15) Yamagata S. [Diagnosis of gastritis.] Iji Shinpo. 1961; 1916: 5–16. (In Japanese.)

16) Article reporting on the gastritis symposium held at the 3rd Congress of the Japan Gastroenterological Endoscopy Society. Gastroenterol Endosc. 1961–1962; 3: 183–240. (In Japanese.)

17) Yoshitani K. [Study about gastritis.] Gastroenterol Endosc. 1961–1962; 3: 260–288. (In Japanese.)

18) Takemoto T, Mizuno Y. [Gastroscopic diagnosis and gastric biopsy of chronic gastritis.] Gastroenterol Endosc. 1962–1963; 4: 310–320. (In Japanese.)

19) Nagai M. [Study about chronic gastritis diagnosis: Focusing especially on images of granular mucosa.] Gastroenterol Endosc. 1962–1963; 4: 253–269. (In Japanese.)

20) Siurala M, Vuorinen Y. Follow-up studies of patients with superficial gastritis and patients with a normal gastric mucosa. Acta Med Scand. 1963; 173: 45–52.

21) Ichioka S. [Endoscopic supplement to chronic gastritis.] Nippon Shokakibyo Gakkai Zasshi. 1964; 61: 785–809. (In Japanese.)

22) Shiraishi H. [Clinical study about follow-ups of chronic gastritis — centering around gastrocamera and gastric biopsy findings.] Gastroenterol Endosc. 1964–1965; 6: 230–246. (In Japanese.)

23) Toyoda S. [Study about gastrocamera images of atrophic gastritis.] Gastroenterol Endosc. 1965; 7: 296–317. (In Japanese.)

24) Umeda N. [Study on chronic gastritis: Clinical and experimental researches centering around atrophic gastritis.] Nippon Shokakibyo Gakkai Zasshi. 1965; 62: 985–1003. (In Japanese.)

25) Muto F. [Study about endoscopic diagnosis of chronic gastritis — centering around especially investigation with gastric biopsy and long-term follow-up cases.] Gastroenterol Endosc. 1967; 9: 372–394. (In Japanese.)

26) Hirafuku I. [Histopathological images of chronic gastritis — focusing on relationship with clinical aspects.] I to Cho (Stomach Intest). 1967; 2: 1257–1264. (In Japanese.)

27) Kimura K, Takemoto T. An endoscopic recognition of the atrophic border and its significance in chronic gastritis. Endoscopy. 1969; 1 (3): 87–96.

28) Oshima H. [Memory of Dr. Schindler and the path he walked.] Gastroenterol Endosc. 1969; 11: 287–295. (In Japanese.)

29) Furuya K. [Supplement to clinical and histopathological knowledge of erosive gastritis observed in resected ulcers.] Nippon Shokakibyo Gakkai Zasshi. 1970; 67: 1115–1126. (In Japanese.)

30) Ariga K (ed). [Clinical Internal Medicine Encyclopedia Vol. 4 — Digestive Disease.] Tokyo: Kanehara Shuppan, 1970. (In Japanese.)

31) Kimura K. Chronological transition of the fundic-pyloric border determined by stepwise biopsy of the lesser and greater curvatures of the stomach. Gastroenterology. 1972; 63: 584–592.

32) Whitehead R, Truelove SC, Gear MW. The histological diagnosis of chronic gastritis in fibreoptic gastroscope biopsy specimens. J Clin Pathol. 1972; 25: 1–11.

33) Takase Y. [An endoscopic and biopsy study on chronic gastritis (I): atrophic gastritis.] Nippon Shokakibyo Gakkai Zasshi. 1973; 70: 99–106. (In Japanese.)

34) Takase Y. [An endoscopic and biopsy study on chronic gastritis (II): criteria for atrophic gastritis by endoscopic examination with light-guide fiber gastroscope.] Nippon Shokakibyo Gakkai Zasshi. 1973; 70: 107–116. (In Japanese.)

35) Strickland RG, Mackay IR. A reappraisal of the nature and significance of chronic atrophic gastritis. Am J Dig Dis. 1973; 18: 426–440.

36) Sada H. [Study of so-called verrucous erosive gastritis.] Gastroenterol Endosc. 1974; 16: 365–385. (In Japanese.)

37) Takasu S, Inui Y. [A report of 100 cases of gastritis verrucosa and their long-term follow-up.] Gastroenterol Endosc. 1974; 16: 763–776. (In Japanese.)

38) Yokoyama I. [Clinical study on endoscopic diagnosis of intestinal metaplasia.] Gastroenterol Endosc. 1975; 17: 65–75. (In Japanese.)

39) Takemoto T (EIC); Takezoe K, Kimura K (ed secs). [Overview of Gastrointestinal Endoscopy Diagnostics Vol. 3: Stomach (1) — Normal Stomach/Gastritis/Erosion.] Tokyo: Igaku-Shoin, 1976. (In Japanese.)

40) Senoo T. [Clinical and endoscopic study of gastric erosion.] Gastroenterol Endosc. 1979; 21: 312–328. (In Japanese.)

41) Yamamura Y (ed supv); Hosoda S, Ichioka S (ed cmte mbrs). [Atlas of Clinical Internal Medicine Vol. 17: Digestive Tract (2-A).] Tokyo: Medical View, 1981. (In Japanese.)

42) Haruma K. [Clinical study on the characteristics of atrophic gastritis in gastric polyp cases.] Hiroshima J Med Sci. 1981: 30: 399–418. (In Japanese.)

43) Yoshii T. [Pathology of the Stomach — Focusing on Interpretation of Histological Images.] Tokyo: Igaku Tosho Shuppan, 1973. (In Japanese.)

44) Sano R. [Clinical Pathology of Gastric Disease.] Tokyo: Igaku Shoin, 1974. (In Japanese.)

45) Warren JR, Marshall B. Unidentified curved bacilli on gastric epithelium in active chronic gastritis. Lancet, 1983; 1 (8336): 1273–1275.

46) Fukushima T, Tsumaru S, Hirata K, et al. [Decrease in somatostatin in the antral mucosa in duodenal ulcer cases.] Nippon Shokakibyo Gakkai Zasshi. 1983; 80: 1105–1110. (In Japanese.)

47) McCormack TT, Sims J, Eyre-Brook I, et al. Gastric lesions in portal hypertension: Inflammatory gastritis or congestive gastropathy? Gut. 1985; 26: 1226–1232.

48) Ihamäki T, Kekki M, Sipponen P, et al. The sequelae and course of chronic gastritis during a 30- to 34-year bioptic follow-up study. Scand J Gastroenterol. 1985; 20: 485–491.

49) Takemoto T. [Chronic gastritis.] Nihon Naika Gakkai Zasshi. 1985; 74: 867–879. (In Japanese.)

50) Kato Y, Kuga H, Harada T. [A clinical study of longitudinal linear redness on the gastric mucosa.] Gastroenterol Endosc. 1985; 27: 362–369. (In Japanese.)

51) Sakita T. [An essay on chronic gastritis.] Gastroenterol Endosc. 1986; 28: 172–181. (In Japanese.)

52) Takemoto T, Shimada M. [Definition and classification of chronic gastritis.] Clinical Gastroenterology. 1987; 2: 7–19. (In Japanese.)

53) Corbishley CM, Saverymuttu SH and Maxwell JD: Use of endoscopic biopsy for diagnosing congestive gastropathy. J Clin Pathol. 1988; 41: 1187–1190.

54) Correa P. Chronic gastritis: A clinico-pathological classification. Am J Gastroenterol. 1988; 83: 504–509.

55) Tytgat GN. The Sydney System: endoscopic division — endoscopic appearances in gastritis/duodenitis. J Gastroenterol Hepatol. 1991; 6: 223–234.

56) Haruma K, Sumii K, Yoshihara M, et al. Gastric mucosa in female patients with fundic glandular polyps. J Clin Gastroenterol. 1991; 13: 565–569.

57) Misiewicz JJ. The Sydney System: a new classification of gastritis. J Gastroenterol Hepatol. 1991; 6: 207–208.

58) Haruma K, Okamato S, Sumii K, et al. *Helicobacter pylori* infection and gastroduodenal disease: a comparison of endoscopic findings, histology, and urease test data. Hiroshima J Med Sci. 1992; 41: 65–70.

59) Saito Y, Saito K, Nakahara A. [Redness observed in endoscopy and histopathological investigation into superficial gastritis.] Gastroenterol Endosc. 1992; 34: 39–47. (In Japanese.)

60) Imura H, Ogata E, Takahisa F, et al. [The Latest Overview of Internal Medicine Vol. 41 — Gastritis.] Tokyo: Nakayama Shoten, 1993. (In Japanese.)

61) Haruma K, Yoshihara M, Sumii K, et al. Gastric acid secretion, serum pepsinogen I, and serum gastrin in Japanese with gastric hyperplastic polyps or polypoid-type early gastric carcinoma. Scand J Gastroenterol. 1993; 28: 633–637.

62) Whitehead R. The classification of chronic gastritis: Current status. J Clin Gastroenterol. 1995; 21 (Suppl 1): 131–134.

63) Kato M, Nishikawa K, Katagiri M, et al. [Classification of gastritis.] GI Research. 1995; 3: 349–356. (In Japanese.)

64) Kato M, Asaka M, Kudoh M, et al. Evaluation of endoscopic characteristics in a new gastritis

classification system. Dig Endosc. 1995; 7: 363–371.

65) Maruyama T. [Investigation of gastric mucosal lesions accompanied by portal hypertension.] Nippon Shokakibyo Gakkai Zasshi. 1995; 92: 1121–1132. (In Japanese.)

66) Haruma K, Komoto K, Kawaguchi H, et al. Pernicious anemia and *Helicobacter pylori* infection in Japan: evaluation in a country with a high prevalence of infection. Am J Gastroenterol. 1995; 90: 1107–1110.

67) 10th Meeting for Gastritis Study. [Classification of gastritis: revised tentative proposal from the Meeting for Gastritis Study.] Ther Res.1995; 16 (10): 37–41. (In Japanese.)

68) Dixon MF, Genta RM, Yardley JH, et al. Classification and grading of gastritis: the updated Sydney system — International Workshop on the Histopathology of Gastritis, Houston, 1994. Am J Surg Pathol. 1996; 20: 1161–1181.

69) Fukuchi S (ed). [Issues of Gastritis Research.] Tokyo: Kokusai Isho Shuppan, 1996. (In Japanese.)

70) Kawaguchi H, Haruma K, Komoto K, et al. *Helicobacter pylori* infection is the major risk factor for atrophic gastritis. Am J Gastroenterol. 1996; 91: 959–962.

71) Shimoda T, Nakanishi Y, Yoshino T. [Histological classification of chronic gastritis: its historical transition.] I to Cho (Stomach Intest). 1998; 33: 1073–1078.

72) Komoto K, Haruma K, Kamada T, et al. *Helicobacter pylori* infection and gastric neoplasia: Correlations with histological gastritis and tumor histology. Am J Gastroenterol. 1998; 93: 1271–1276.

73) Mihara M, Haruma K, Kamada T, et al. The role of endoscopic findings for the diagnosis of *Helicobacter pylori* infection: evaluation in a country with high prevalence of atrophic gastritis. Helicobacter. 1999; 4: 40–48.

74) Haruma K, Mihara M, Okamoto E, et al. Eradication of *Helicobacter pylori* increases gastric acidity in patients with atrophic gastritis of the corpus-evaluation of 24-h pH monitoring. Aliment Pharmacol Ther. 1999; 13: 155–162.

75) Haruma K, Kamada T, Kawaguchi H, et al. Effect of age and *Helicobacter pylori* infection on gastric acid secretion. J Gastroenterol Hepatol. 2000; 15: 277–283.

76) Kaminishi M, Yamaguchi H, Nomura S, et al. Endoscopic classification of chronic gastritis based on a pilot study by the research society for gastritis. Dig Endosc. 2002; 14: 138–151.

77) Ito M, Haruma K, Kamada T, et al. *Helicobacter pylori* eradication therapy improves atrophic gastritis and intestinal metaplasia: a 5-year prospective study of patients with atrophic gastritis. Aliment Pharmacol Ther. 2002; 16: 1449–1456.

78) Rugge M, Genta RM; OLGA-Group. Staging gastritis: an international proposal. Gastroenterology. 2005; 129: 1807–1808.

79) Rugge M, Genta RM. Staging and grading of chronic gastritis. Hum Pathol. 2005; 36: 228–233.

80) Sipponen P. Chronic gastritis in former times and now. Helicobacter. 2007; 12 (Suppl 2): 16–21.

81) Kamada T, Tanaka A, Yamanaka Y, et al. Nodular gastritis with *Helicobacter pylori* infection is strongly associated with diffuse-type gastric cancer in young patients. Dig Endosc. 2007; 19: 180–184.

82) Tanaka A, Kamada T, Inoue K, et al. Histological evaluation of patients with gastritis at high risk of developing gastric cancer using a conventional index. Pathol Res Pract. 2011; 207: 354–358.

83) Nomura S, Terao S, Adachi K, et al. Endoscopic diagnosis of gastric mucosal activity and inflammation. Dig Endosc. 2013; 25: 136–146.

84) Kato M, Terao S, Adachi K, et al. Changes in endoscopic findings of gastritis after cure of *H. pylori* infection: multicenter prospective trial. Dig Endosc. 2013; 25: 264–273.

85) Nomura S, Ida K, Terao S, et al. Endoscopic diagnosis of gastric mucosal atrophy: multicenter prospective study. Dig Endosc. 2014 ; 26 : 709-719.

Chapter 2

Endoscopic Findings

of Gastritis

Chapter 2   Endoscopic Findings of Gastritis

1. Introduction

Tomoari Kamada

Chronic gastritis is inflammation and atrophic change of the stomach accompanied by *Helicobacter pylori* (*H. pylori*) infection. Chronic gastritis can lead to a variety of intragastric diseases such as gastric cancer, peptic ulcers, mucosa associated lymphoid tissue (MALT) lymphoma, and foveolar hyperplastic polyps, as well as extragastric diseases such as immune thrombocytopenic purpura, iron-deficiency anemia, and chronic urticaria. To treat gastritis and prevent these diseases, especially gastric cancer, eradication treatment of *H. pylori*-infected gastritis is critical. Consequently, this was brought under the coverage of the Japanese health insurance system on February 21, 2013.

When humans are infected with *H. pylori*, a chronic gastritis condition called chronic active gastritis develops in which acute inflammation and chronic inflammation coexist. From a histological point of view, this chronic inflammation of the gastric mucosa is called *Helicobacter pylori*-infected gastritis. Diagnosis of this disease requires upper gastrointestinal endoscopy. This is a disease concept independent of chronic gastritis — the term generally used in actual clinical practice in Japan; it is a disease that requires that eradication treatment of *H. pylori* be prioritized.

To simplify diagnosis of endoscopic findings of gastritis in upper gastrointestinal endoscopy, *H. pylori* infection is separated into three phases. The Kyoto Classification of Gastritis incorporating these three phases is shown in **Table 1**.

 ***H. pylori*-uninfected gastric mucosa = Normal stomach**

This is a condition in which the gastric mucosa has not been infected with *H. pylori* and in which there is no histological gastritis such as atrophy, neutrophil infiltration, and intestinal metaplasia. In endoscopy, a regular arrangement of collective venules (RAC) present in the subepithelial mucosa is observed from the lower corpus to the lesser curvature of the angulus[1]. The appearance of the gastric mucosa is relatively smooth and glossy, the degree of viscosity is very low, and straight folds can be seen running along the greater curvature of the corpus. Incidental findings in the stomach — such as a fundic gland polyp, hematin attachment, and red streak in the antrum and corpus — are sometimes recognized.

Chapter 2 Endoscopic Findings of Gastritis

Table 1   Kyoto Classification of Gastritis

Region	Endoscopic findings	*H. pylori* infected	*H. pylori* uninfected	After *H. pylori* eradication
Entire gastric mucosa	Atrophy	○	×	○-×
	Diffuse redness	○	×	×
	Foveolar-hyperplastic polyp	○	×	○-×
	Map-like redness	×	×	○
	Xanthoma	○	×	○
	Hematin	△	○	○
	Red streak	△	○	○
	Intestinal metaplasia	○	×	○-△
	Mucosal swelling	○	×	×
	Patchy redness	○	○	○
	Depressive erosion	○	○	○
Corpus	Enlarged fold, tortuous fold	○	×	×
	Sticky mucus	○	×	×
Corpus to fornix	Fundic gland polyp	×	○	○
	Spotty redness	○	×	△-×
	Multiple white and flat elevated lesions	△	○	○
Lesser curvature of lower corpus to Lesser curvature of angulus	Regular arrangement of collecting venules (RAC)	×	○	×-△
antrum	Nodularity	○	×	△-×
	Raised erosion	△	○	○

○: Frequently observed   ×: Not observed △: Sometimes observed

Note: For the regions of endoscopic findings, refer to **Table 2**

2 Currently *H. pylori*-infected gastric mucosa = Chronic active gastritis (CAG)[2]

H. pylori-infected gastric mucosa is marked by the presence of mononuclear cell infiltration and neutrophil infiltration. In addition, atrophy of the proper gastric gland and intestinal metaplasia caused by chronic changes are also observed. Endoscopic findings include spotty redness or diffuse redness from the corpus to the fornix, disappearance of RAC, atrophy (atypical vascular pattern or faded mucosa), abnormal folds (enlarged, tortuous, or vanished), mucosal swelling,

Table 2　Regions of endoscopic findings

Endoscopic findings	See	Regions					
		Fornix	Upper corpus	Middle corpus	Lower corpus	Angulus	Antrum
Atrophy	p.30 – 32						
Diffuse redness	p.38 – 42						
Foveolar-hyperplastic polyp	p.57 – 59						
Map-like redness	p.88 – 90						
Xanthoma	p.60 – 62						
Hematin	p.77 – 78						
Red streak	p.71 – 74						
Intestinal metaplasia	p.33 – 37						
Mucosal swelling	p.46 – 48						
Patchy redness	p.83 – 87						
Depressive erosion	p.63 – 65						
Enlarged folds, tortuous folds	p.49 – 51						
Sticky mucus	–						
Fundic gland polyp	p.68 – 70						
Spotty redness	p.43 – 45						
Multiple white and flat elevated lesions	p.91 – 93						
Regular arrangement of collecting venules (RAC)	p.66 – 67				(Lesser curvature)	(Lesser curvature)	
Nodularity	p.52 – 56						
Raised erosion	p.75 – 76						

intestinal metaplasia, foveolar hyperplastic polyp, xanthoma, nodularity (nodular changes), and sticky mucus. Diagnosis of atrophic gastritis, metaplastic gastritis (intestinal metaplasia), enlarged fold gastritis, and nodular gastritis is an extreme important to require accurate endoscopic diagnosis.

1) Atrophic gastritis and metaplastic gastritis

The conventional classification of gastritis used in Japan — the Kimura-Takemoto Classification[3] (Fig. 2 on page 11) — classifies the extent of atrophic gastritis in the corpus based on endoscopic findings. This classification system is well established in Japan and remains important to this day in assessing the risk of gastric cancer and the state of gastric acid secretion. In atrophic gastritis, the folds in the lesser curvature of the corpus disappear while the gastric mucosa becomes thinner, and endoscopic atrophic borders can be confirmed in findings of faded mucosa accompanied by reticulated and dendritic vascular patterns. This is best diagnosed using the indigo carmine contrast method together with image enhanced endoscopy (IEE) such as Narrow Band Imaging (NBI) or Autofluorescence Imaging (AFI)[4]. Metaplastic gastritis refers to the condition in which atrophic changes occur in the gastric mucosa, accompanied by intestinal metaplasia. In such an environment, *H. pylori* itself may no longer be able to survive and as a consequence may not be detected. In endoscopic observation, multiple white and flat elevated lesions of varying sizes can be seen in the background of atrophic gastric mucosa. In NBI magnifying endoscopy, light blue crests (LBC) have recently come into popular use as an index for diagnosis of intestinal metaplasia[5].

2) Enlarged fold gastritis and nodular gastritis

Diseases that cause enlarged gastric folds include neoplastic diseases such as gastric cancer and malignant lymphoma and non-neoplastic diseases caused by hyperplasia of gastric foveolar epithelial cells. Those that exhibit non-neoplastic enlargement of folds are called enlarged fold gastritis. Caused by *H. pylori* infection, enlarged fold gastritis features thickening of the mucosa — caused by hyperproliferation of epithelial cells and hyperplasia of foveolar epithelium — along with inflammatory cell infiltration in the corpus. Studies have shown that in cases in which the width of the folds is greater than 7 mm, the risk of gastric cancer — especially diffuse type gastric cancer in the corpus — is 35.5 times higher than in cases with a folds width of less than 4 mm[6]. Reports also indicate that eradication of *H. pylori* can significantly improve outcomes in cases of enlarged fold gastritis[7].

Nodular gastritis is a type of gastritis characterized endoscopically by raised lesions with a uniform granular or nodular texture resembling gooseflesh that are distributed in the region from the antrum to the angulus[8]. Commonly seen in young women, it is also found frequently in *H. pylori*-infected young adults, as well as in children[9]. Nodular gastritis is often associated with peptic ulcers and gastric cancer, and is tconsidered a high risk factor for undifferentiated gastric cancer[10].

 Previously *H. pylori*-infected gastric mucosa (natural disappearance of *H. pylori* after eradication or advanced atrophy) = Chronic inactive gastritis (CIG)[2]

Although neurotrophic infiltration promptly disappears after *H. pylori* has been eradicated, mononuclear cell infiltration often remains. This finding usually indicates a previous infection when spotty redness or diffuse redness in the region from the corpus to the fornix has disappeared (RAC may be partially observed), the atrophic border becomes unclear, the mucosa looks smooth and glossy, and the folds in the greater curvature of the corpus appear normal. Atrophic mucosa (atypical vascular pattern or faded mucosa) is recognized endoscopically. It should be noted that the disappearance of diffuse redness often results in the appearance of map-like redness in the corpus and antrum.

Watanabe et al.[11] studied various endoscopic findings that would be able to predict *H. pylori* infections and reported that RAC, hematin attachment, fundic gland polyps, atrophic changes, and map-like redness were all helpful in predicting status of *H. pylori* infection.

Changes in the gastric mucosa caused by drugs

Drug-induced gastritis is a form of gastritis that can develop independently of *H. pylori* infection. Among the drugs that can damage the stomach, representative drugs are antithrombotic agents such as aspirin, typical nonsteroidal anti-inflammatory drugs, and proton pump inhibitors. Findings observed that show aspirin usage include patchy redness, depressive erosion, spotty redness, and hematin. In cases of long-term use of proton pump inhibitors, cobblestone mucosa and multiple white and flat elevated lesion are frequently observed and flat in the region from the fornix to the corpus.

References

1) Yagi K, Nakamura A and Sekine A : Characteristic endoscopic and magnified endoscopic findings in the normal stomach without *Helicobacter pylori* infection. J Gastroenterol Hepatol 2002 ; 17 : 39-45
2) Dixon MF, Genta RM, Yardley JH, et al : Classification and grading of gastritis. The updated Sydney System. International Workshop on the Histopathology of Gastritis, Houston 1994. Am J Surg Pathol 1996 ; 20 : 1161-1181
3) Kimura K and Takemoto T : An endoscopic recognition of atrophic border and its significance in chronic gastritis. Endoscopy 1969 ; 1 : 87-97
4) Hanaoka N, Uedo N, Shiotani A, et al : Autofluorescence imaging for predicting development of metachronous gastric cancer after *Helicobacter pylori* eradication. J Gastroenterol Hepatol 2010 ; 25 : 1844-1849
5) Uedo N, Ishihara R, Iishi H, et al : A new method of diagnosing gastric intestinal metaplasia : narrow-band imaging with magnifying endoscopy. Endoscopy 2006 ; 38 : 819-824
6) Nishibayashi H, Kanayama S, Kiyohara T, et al : *Helicobacter pylori*-induced enlarged-fold gastritis is associated with increased mutagenicity of gastric juice, increased oxidative DNA damage, and an increased risk of gastric carcinoma. J Gastroenterol Hepatol 2003 ; 18 : 1384-1391
7) Yasunaga Y, Shinomura Y, Kanayama S, et al : Improved fold width and increased acid secretion after eradication of the organism in *Helicobacter pylori* associated enlarged fold gastritis. Gut 1994 ; 35 : 1571-1574
8) Takemoto T, Mizuno Y. : [Gastroscopic diagnosis and biopsy of chronic gastritis.] Gastroenterol Endosc 1962; 4: 310-320 (In Japanese)
9) Miyamoto M, Haruma K, Yoshihara M, et al : Nodular gastritis in adults is caused by *Helicobacter pylori* infection. Dig Dis Sci 2003 ; 48 : 968-975
10) Kamada T, Tanaka A, Yamanaka Y, et al : Nodular gastritis with *Helicobacter pylori* infection is strongly associated with diffuse-type gastric cancer in young patients. Dig Endosc 2007 ; 19 : 180-184
11) Watanabe K, Nagata N, Nakashima R, et al : Predictive findings for *Helicobacter pylori*-uninfected, -infected and -eradicated gastric mucosa : validation study. World J Gastroenterol 2013 ; 19 : 4374-4379

Chapter 2 Endoscopic Findings of Gastritis
2. Specific Discussions
1 Atrophy

Kazunari Murakami

Description ▶▶ Page 32

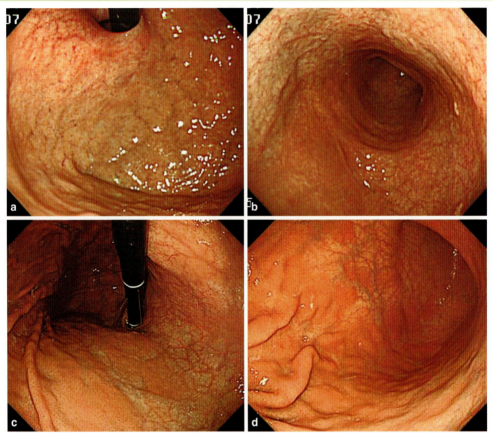

Fig. 1 Typical images of atrophic gastritis

a: Obvious vascular pattern is recognized in the cardia.
b: Corpus viewed from above.
c: Lesser curvature of the angulus viewed from below.
d: Atrophic border in the lower corpus.

• Equipment used (Pages 30–31)
 Endoscopes: GIF-Q240, GIF-Q260 (Olympus)
 Light source: EVIS LUCERA CLV-260SL (Olympus)

2. Specific Discussions • 31

Fig. 2 Improvement in endoscopic atrophy

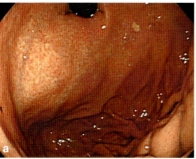
Before eradication

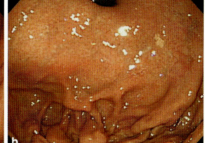
15 months after eradication

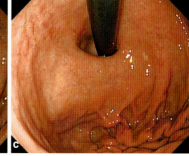
5 years after eradication

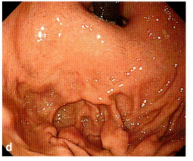
7 years after eradication

a: Male, 71 years old. Before eradication. The atrophic border goes beyond the cardia and expands towards the fornix.
b: 15 months after eradication. Although mucosal redness and spotty redness have decreased, the atrophic border seems to be about the same as it was prior to eradication.
c: 5 years after eradication. The atrophic border that went beyond the fornix side has receded to the corpus side and the atrophy around the cardia has disappeared.
d: 7 years after eradication: The atrophy in the fornix and atrophic border can no longer be seen. The atrophic border has continued to improve with the passage of time and is much reduced compared to prior to the eradication.

Fig. 3 Improvement in histologic atrophy

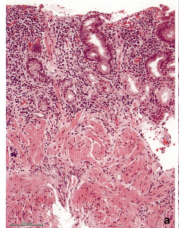
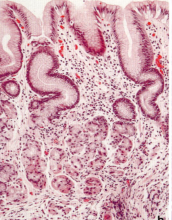
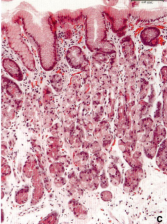

Before eradication　　　6 months after eradication　　　5 years after eradication

Male, 62 years old. Chronic gastritis case. Biopsied tissue from the greater curvature of the corpus.
a: Advanced acute and chronic inflammatory cell infiltration can be seen before eradication. Fundic gland has decreased significantly due to atrophy.
b: 6 months after eradication. Inflammatory cell infiltration shows noticeable improvement. Some fundic gland can be seen, but the amount is small and atrophy can be observed.
c: 5 years after eradication. The chronic inflammatory cell infiltration has decreased significantly. The amount of fundic gland tissue has noticeably increased and there is less atrophy.

Atrophy

Description

Endoscopic atrophy is assessed by observing images of vascular patterns. To observe the degree and extent of the atrophy, the site must be adequately insufflated **(Fig. 1)**. In 1969, Kimura and Takemoto classified atrophic gastritis. With this, atrophy extends from the pyloric region and is classified into six grades — C-1, C-2, C-3, O-1, O-2, and O-3 — according to the size of the area (Fig. 2 on page 11). "C" stands for closed and "O" for open. When the atrophy is continuous from the cardia to the pylorus, it is called an open type. When it is not continuous, it is classified as a closed type. In terms of histology, the decrease of proper gastric glands on the gastric mucosa is called atrophy **(Fig. 3)**. This is generally thought to be caused by accelerated shedding of epithelial cells due to *H. pylori* infection and inflammation.

It is rare to find atrophy in patients who have not been infected with *H. pylori*. However, in Type A gastritis patients, atrophy is seen in the corpus, but not in the pylorus.

After eradication, atrophy is significantly improved in terms of histology. Nevertheless, there are many cases in which no improvement is recognized endoscopically **(Fig. 2)** (the vascular patterns are the same before and after the eradication).

References

1) Murakami K, Kodama M, Sato R, et al : *Helicobacter pylori* eradication and associated changes in the gastric mucosa. Expert Rev Anti Infect Ther   2005 ; 3 : 757-764
2) Kodama M, Murakami K, Okimoto T, et al : Ten-year prospective follow-up of histological changes at five points on the gastric mucosa as recommended by the updated Sydney system after *Helicobacter pylori* eradication. J Gastroenterol   2012 ; 47 : 394-403
3) Ito M, Haruma K, Kamada T, et al : *Helicobacter pylori* eradication therapy improves atrophic gastritis and intestinal metaplasia : a 5-year prospective study of patients with atrophic gastritis. Aliment Pharmacol Ther   2002 ; 16 : 1449-1456
4) Toyokawa T, Suwaki K, Miyake Y, et al : Eradication of *Helicobacter pylori* infection improved gastric mucosal atrophy and prevented progression of intestinal metaplasia, especially in the elderly population : a long-term prospective cohort study. J Gastroenterol Hepatol   2010 ; 25 : 544-547
5) Vannella L, Lahner E, Bordi C, et al : Reversal of atrophic body gastritis after *H. pylori* eradication at long-term follow-up. Dig Liver Dis   2011 ; 43 : 295-299

2 Intestinal metaplasia

Masashi Kawamura

📖 Description ▶▶ Page 37

Fig. 1   Endoscopic intestinal metaplasia exhibiting grayish white elevation found in the antrum of an *H. pylori*-positive patient

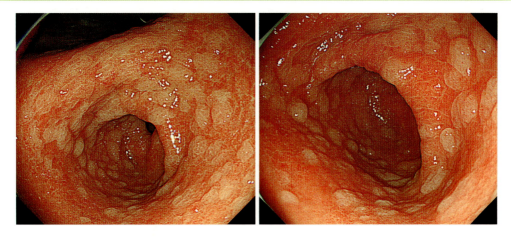

Fig. 2   Endoscopic image of indigo carmine sprayed intestinal metaplasia exhibiting grayish white elevation found in the antrum of an *H. pylori*-positive patient

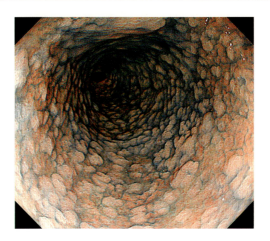

- Equipment used (Pages 33–36)
  Endoscopes: GIF-H260 (Figs. 2, 4, 5), GIF-H260Z (Figs. 1, 3, 6–9) (Olympus)
  Light source: EVIS LUCERA CLV-260SL (Olympus)

34 ● Chapter 2 Endoscopic Findings of Gastritis

Fig. 3 Grayish white elevation found in the region from the antrum to the corpus of an *H. pylori*-positive patient

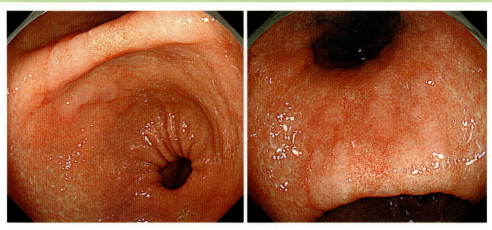

Fig. 4 Grayish white mucosa found in the region from the antrum to the corpus of an *H. pylori*-positive patient

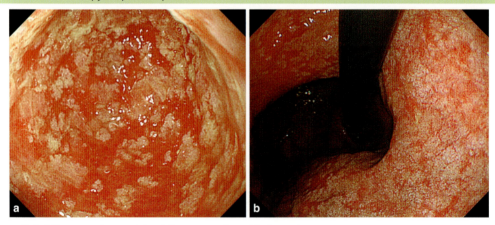

a: Pellet-like granular grayish white mucosa found in the antrum.
b: Intragastric bile reflux is observed, and the grayish white mucosa extends as far as the corpus.

Fig. 5 Endoscopic intestinal metaplasia exhibiting roof slate type grayish white mucosa found in the antrum of an *H. pylori*-positive patient

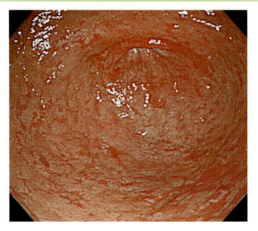

Fig. 6 Intestinal metaplasia found in the corpus of an *H. pylori*-positive patient

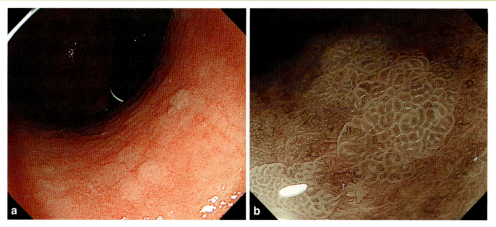

a: Specific intestinal metaplasia found in the corpus of an *H. pylori*-positive patient.
b: Light blue crests (LBCs) can be seen on the grayish white elevation in Narrow Band Imaging (NBI) magnifying observation. [Structure Enhancement: B8; Color Enhancement: 1]

Fig. 7 LBCs found in chronic atrophic gastritis accompanied by *H. pylori* infection

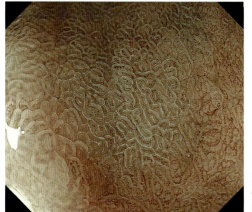

LBCs can be seen in areas other than the grayish white elevation. [Structure Enhancement: B8; Color Enhancement: 1]

Fig. 8 NBI magnified endoscopic image of a grayish white elevation found in an *H. pylori*-positive patient

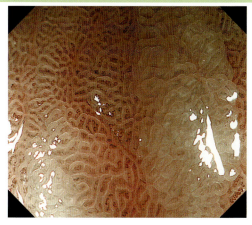

White opaque substance (WOS) is found in interfoveolar regions that correspond to the grayish white elevation. [Structure Enhancement: B8; Color Enhancement: 1]

36 ● Chapter 2 Endoscopic Findings of Gastritis

Fig. 9　Small white elevation found in a non-atrophic area (fornix)

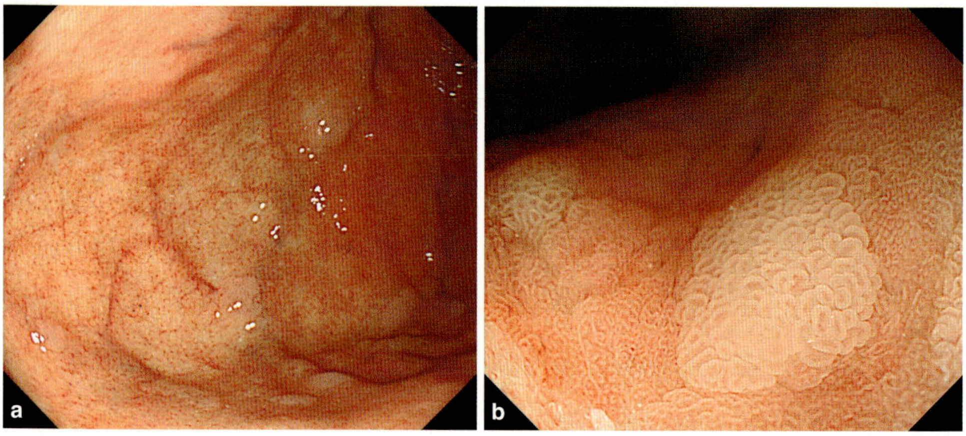

a: Small white elevation found in a non-atrophic area (fornix) after *H. pylori* eradication. Biopsy shows hyperplasia in the foveolar epithelium. Small white elevations such as this are sometimes found in patients who have taken proton pump inhibitors (PPIs).

b: Orderly papillary structure is observed in a magnification close-up image.

Intestinal Metaplasia

 Description

Endoscopic findings of intestinal metaplasia are observed as grayish white mucosa, which is part of the mucosal atrophy associated with chronic gastritis caused by *H. pylori* infection. The most typical images of endoscopic intestinal metaplasia are grayish white flat elevations usually found in the pyloric antrum (specific intestinal metaplasia [Yokoyama, Takemoto, et al[1]]) (**Figs. 1 & 2**). Specific intestinal metaplasia is found in many different cases, progressing at the same rate as atrophic gastritis (**Fig. 3**).

In some cases, endoscopic intestinal metaplasia also shows grayish white mucosa that does not exhibit the typical flat elevation. These are referred to as roof slate type, scattered rice grain type, or pellet-like granular type (**Figs. 4 & 5**). Since endoscopic intestinal metaplasia is also observed in gastric mucosa after *H. pylori* eradication, this finding is seen not only in *H. pylori*-infected cases, but also in cases previously infected with *H. pylori*.

The grayish white mucosa observed endoscopically is a useful endoscopic finding for intestinal metaplasia because histological intestinal metaplasia is frequently found in biopsies. However, because histological intestinal metaplasia is not seen only in grayish white mucosa[2], it is problematic to rely solely on endoscopy to diagnose all types — including complete and incomplete types — of histological intestinal metaplasia.

Recent studies have found that light blue crests (LBCs) observed in Narrow Band Imaging (NBI) — a type of image enhanced endoscopy (IEE) — around the gastric mucosal epithelium are related to histological intestinal metaplasia[3] (**Figs. 6 & 7**). When grayish white mucosa is observed with NBI, a white opaque substance (WOS)[4] is sometimes found in interfoveolar regions of the gastric mucosa (**Fig. 8**). It is to be hoped that in the future a reliable diagnostic method will be established for endoscopic intestinal metaplasia — for example, chromoendoscopy using methylene blue dye[5].

It is also important to differentiate flat elevated lesions such as gastric adenoma from grayish white endoscopic intestinal metaplasia. Specific intestinal metaplasia is distinguished by frequent occurrence in the antrum, while small white elevations caused by foveolar epithelial hyperplasia are sometimes observed in endoscopic non-atrophic regions from the fornix to the corpus (**Fig. 9**). These small white elevations are often seen in patients who have taken proton pump inhibitors (PPIs) and are distinguished by their small size and sparse distribution in non-atrophic mucosa.

References

1) Yokoyama I, Takemoto T, Kimura K: [Endoscopic diagnosis of intestinal metaplasia.] I to Cho (Stomach Intest) 1971; 6: 869–874
2) Kaminishi M, Yamaguchi H, Nomura S, et al. : Endoscopic classification of chronic gastritis based on a pilot study by the Research Society for Gastritis. Dig Endosc 2002; 14: 138–151
3) Uedo N, Ishihara R, Iishi H, et al. : A new method of diagnosing gastric intestinal metaplasia: Narrow-band imaging with magnifying endoscopy. Endoscopy 2006; 38: 819–824
4) Yao K, Iwashita A, Tanabe H, et al. : White opaque substance within superficial elevated gastric neoplasia as visualized by magnification endoscopy with narrow-band imaging: a new optical sign for differentiating between adenoma and carcinoma. Gastrointest Endosc 2008; 68: 574–580
5) Suzuki S, Suzuki H, Endo M, et al. : Endoscopic dyeing method for diagnosis of early cancer and intestinal metaplasia of the stomach. Endoscopy 1973; 5: 124–129

3 Diffuse redness

Shuichi Terao

📖 Description ▶▶ Page 42

Fig. 1 Diffuse redness (greater curvature of the corpus)

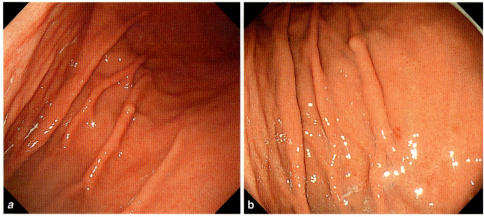

Before eradication   After eradication

Diffuse redness refers to uniform redness with continuous expansion. In this case, diffuse redness is seen over almost the entire field of view of the greater curvature of the corpus. However, it disappears after eradication.

Fig. 2 Diffuse redness (close-up images of the greater curvature of the corpus)

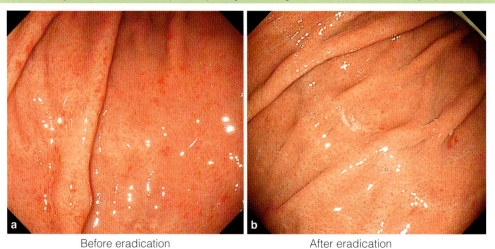

Before eradication   After eradication

Close-up images of the same case as in Fig. 1. Some concurrent spotty redness remains even after eradication.

Fig. 3 Diffuse redness (in the vicinity of the glandular border on the anterior wall of the inferior corpus)

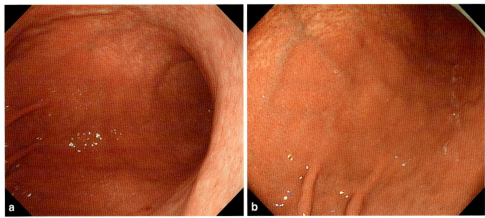

| Before eradication | After eradication |

The same case as shown in Fig. 1. Disappearance and reduction of diffuse redness after *H. pylori* eradication can easily be seen by comparing the atrophic area with the non-atrophic area at the glandular border recognized in the endoscopic view.

Fig. 4 Irregular disappearance and reduction of diffuse redness

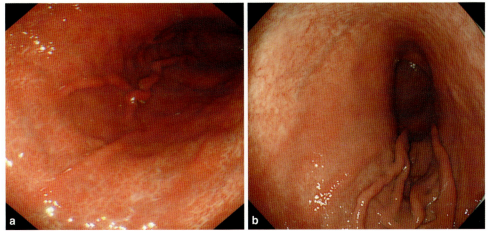

| Before eradication | After eradication |

In some cases, the diffuse redness may not lessen or disappear uniformly after successful *H. pylori* eradication, presenting a characteristic endoscopic image with continuous and gradual reduction of the degree of redness as shown in Fig. 4b.

- Equipment used (Pages 38–41)
  Endoscopes: GIF-H260 (Figs. 1a, 2a, 3a, 6), GIF-H260Z (Figs. 1b, 2b, 3b, 4, 5) (Olympus)
  Light source: EVIS LUCERA CLV-260SL (Olympus)
- Structure Enhancement: B3 (Figs. 1a, 2a, 3a), A1 (Figs. 1b, 2b, 3b, 4)
- Color Enhancement: 0 (Figs. 1–4)

Fig. 5 Close-up images and magnifying NBI images of diffuse redness

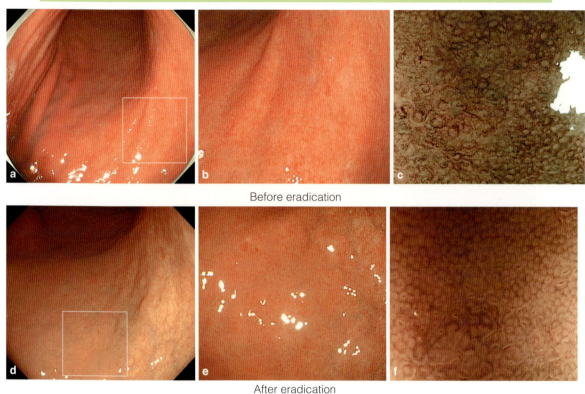

Before eradication

After eradication

Before *H. pylori* eradication (top row: **a–c**) and 3 months after eradication (bottom row: **d–f**).
Distant images (**a, d**): Diffuse redness can be seen throughout the field of view before eradication. It disappears after eradication.
Close-up images (**b, e**): The areas enclosed in the squares in the distant images.
Magnifying NBI images (**c, f**): When the site is observed with NBI before eradication, the glandular structure of the fundic glands looks disordered, glandular density has decreased, and many subepithelial capillaries are visible. After eradication, the glandular openings are restored to their original morphology, glandular density has increased, and fewer capillaries are visible due to the enlarged white zone. [**c**: Structure Enhancement — A3, Color Enhancement — 1; **f**: Structure Enhancement — A1, Color Enhancement — 1]

Fig. 6 Effects of image enhancement

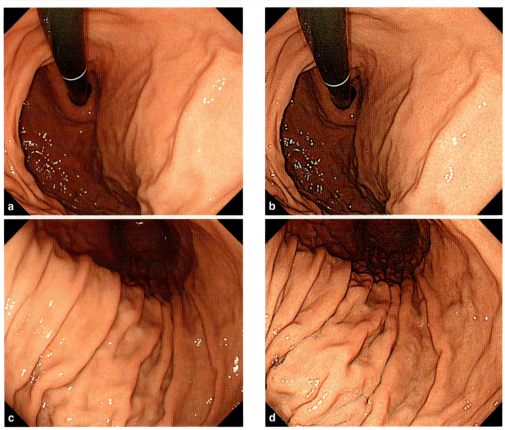

Structure Enhancement: A1;
Color Enhancement: 0

Structure Enhancement: A8;
Color Enhancement: 0

In this case, *H. pylori* IgG antibody was 34 U/mL, PG I was 43.7 ng/mL, PG II was 12.5 ng/mL, and PG I/II was 3.5. The ABC risk assessment corresponded to Group B (^{13}C-UBT 36.5‰). Some enlarged folds and tortuous folds were observed, but there were no findings that showed nodularity, atrophic change, or intestinal metaplasia (C-1). In a case like this, virtually the only basis for diagnosis of *H. pylori* infection would be diffuse redness.

With Structure Enhancement set at A1 (left side: **a**, **c**), diffuse redness can be diagnosed as slightly positive. However, when Structure Enhancement is set at an excessive level (right side: b, d), it can be diagnosed as a finding with many areas of spotty redness. Actually, when we held a meeting to interpret these endoscopic images, one doctor diagnosed it as RAC-positive, *H. pylori* infection suspected.

Diffuse redness

Description

Diffuse redness refers to uniformly reddish mucosa with continuous expansion observed in non-atrophic mucosa mainly in the corpus (**Figs. 1 & 2**). Along with mucosal swelling, diffuse redness is a basic finding for *H. pylori*-infected gastritis (existing infection). It is a finding that shows significant correlation with the degrees of neutrophil infiltration and mononuclear cell infiltration caused by *H. pylori* infection[1,2]. The diffuse redness disappears or decreases after *H. pylori* eradication[3]. While this change occurs relatively quickly and can usually be confirmed as soon as 3 months after eradication (**Fig. 5**), it lasts for a long period of time[4].

In post-eradication endoscopy, the disappearance or reduction of diffuse redness should be actively diagnosed. It is worth noting, however, that assessment of the degree of redness, will be affected by the setting of the endoscope and monitor at each facility. Disappearance and reduction of diffuse redness may occur unevenly in post-eradication endoscopy, resulting in gradations in the degree of redness (**Fig. 4b**). More objective indices — such as comparison between atrophic mucosa and color tones in the vicinity of the glandular border (**Fig. 3b**) — are sometimes observed. Additionally, when the Structure Enhancement setting of the endoscope is set to High, diffuse redness can be observed as an aggregate of small spotty red areas, making it impossible accurate evaluation (**Fig. 6**).

References

1) Ida K, Matsumoto N, Uchiyama K, et al. : [Changes in endoscopic images of gastric mucosa after *Helicobacter pylori* eradication — short-term follow-up cases.] I to Cho (Stomach Intest) 1998; 33: 1115–1121 (In Japanese)
2) Nomura S, Terao S, Adachi K, et al. : Endoscopic diagnosis of gastric mucosal activity and inflammation. Dig Endosc 2013; 25: 136–146
3) Kato M, Terao S, Adachi K, et al. : Changes in endoscopic findings of gastritis after cure of *H. pylori* infection: multicenter prospective trial. Dig Endosc 2013; 25: 264–273
4) Terao S, Nishizawa A, Tamura I, et al: [Investigation into endoscopic images after *H. pylori*-gastritis eradication and comparison of magnifying NBI images immediately after and 10 years after eradication.] Jpn J Gastroenterol 2013; 57: 111–118 (In Japanese)

2. Specific Discussions • 43

4 Spotty redness

Shuichi Terao

📖 Description ▶▶ Page 45

Fig. 1 Spotty redness

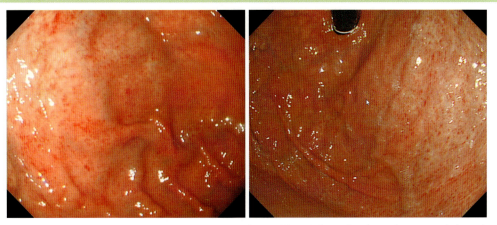

Spotty redness is marked by a relatively even surface with red dots of various shapes and sizes. It is seen in patients infected with *H. pylori* and appears on a background of diffuse redness, typically emerging in the region from the corpus to the fornix.

Fig. 2 Changes in spotty redness after eradication (1)

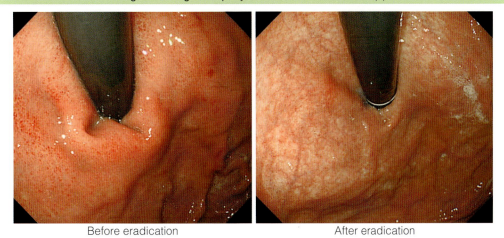

Before eradication | After eradication

Spotty redness often disappears or decreases as a result of *H. pylori* eradication. In this case, disappearance of diffuse redness and reduction of mucosal swelling can also be seen.

• Equipment used (Pages 43–44)
  Endoscope: GIF-H260 (Olympus)
  Light source: EVIS LUCERA CLV-260SL (Olympus)

Fig. 3 Changes in spotty redness after eradication (2)

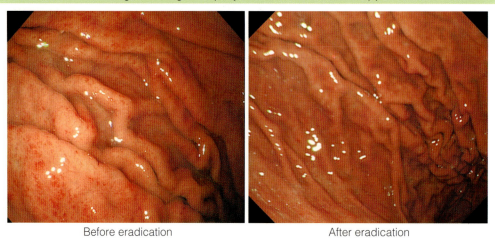

Before eradication — After eradication

When eradication is successful, spotty redness often disappears along with diffuse redness. In this case, enlarged folds and edematous mucosa have also decreased.

Fig. 4 Similar finding seen in portal hypertensive gastropathy

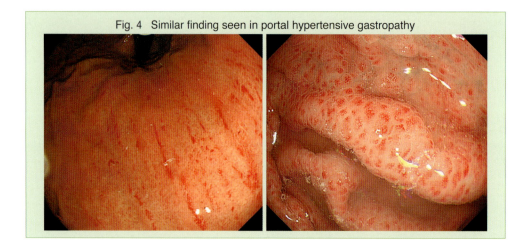

Spotty redness

Description

Spotty redness is marked by irregular red dots of various shapes and sizes. It is seen in patients infected with *H. pylori* (existing infection)[1] and appears on a background of diffuse redness, typically emerging in the region from the corpus to the fornix (**Figs. 1 & 2**). When *H. pylori* eradication is successful, spotty redness often disappears or decreases[2]. In the cases shown in Figs. 2 and **3**, disappearance of diffuse redness, reduction of mucosal swelling, reduction of enlarged folds, and reduction of edematous mucosa are observed simultaneously with the post-eradication disappearance of the spotty redness. It is important to be aware of the fact that findings similar to spotty redness are also observed in portal hypertensive gastropathy, and which are irrelevant to *H. pylori* infection (**Fig. 4**).

Another finding similar to spotty redness, but which needs to be strictly differentiated, is map-like redness. Map-like redness usually appears after *H. pylori* has been successfully eradicated. Unlike spotty redness, map-like redness exhibits various morphologies such as slightly depressed, speckled, patchy patterns and small round depressions (see "18. Map-like redness" below). It is important not to set Structure Enhancement too high when performing endoscopy as this may cause map-like redness to look like multiple aggregates of spotty redness, resulting in incorrect evaluation (Figs. 1–4 were captured with Structure Enhancement A1 and Color Enhancement 0).

References

1) Nomura S, Terao S, Adachi K, et al : Endoscopic diagnosis of gastric mucosal activity and inflammation. Dig Endosc 2013 ; 25 : 136-146
2) Kato M, Terao S, Adachi K, et al : Changes in endoscopic findings of gastritis after cure of *H. pylori* infection : multicenter prospective trial. Dig Endosc 2013 ; 25 : 264-273

5 Mucosal swelling

Takahiro Kato

📖 Description ▶▶ Page 48

Fig. 1　Mucosal swelling not seen in *H. pylori*-uninfected gastric mucosa

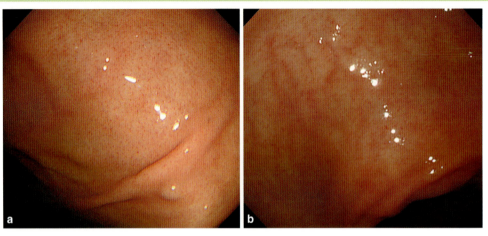

a: Fundic gland mucosa　　b: Pyloric gland mucosa

Fig. 2　Mucosal swelling and swollen areae gastricae (AG) seen in *H. pylori*-infected fundic gland mucosa

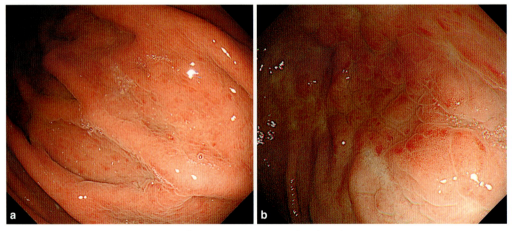

a, b: Mucosal swelling and swollen AG observed in conventional endoscopy

- Equipment used (Pages 46–47)
  Endoscopes: GIF-Q260, GIF-KH260, GIF-H260 (Olympus)
  Light source: EVIS LUCERA CLV-260SL (Olympus)

Fig. 2 Continued from previous page

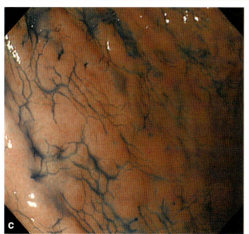

c: Swollen AG visualized with contrast imaging

Fig. 3 Mucosal swelling and swollen areae gastricae (AG) seen in *H. pylori*-infected pyloric gland mucosa

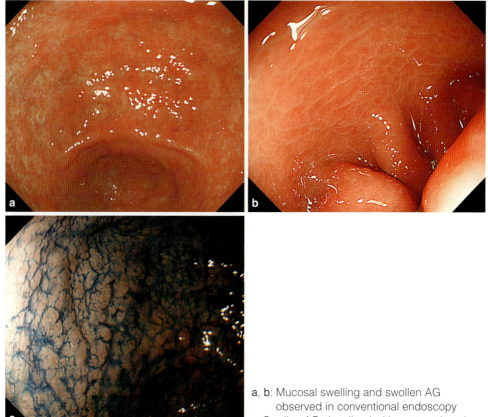

a, b: Mucosal swelling and swollen AG observed in conventional endoscopy
c: Swollen AG visualized with contrast imaging

Fig. 4 Histological finding of mucosal swelling

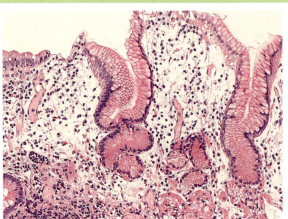

Inflammatory cell infiltration and edema of the mucosa are most noticeable.

Mucosal swelling

Description

Mucosal swelling is not observed in *H. pylori*-uninfected gastric mucosa (**Fig. 1**). It is, however, an important finding in *H. pylori*-infected gastric mucosa (**Figs. 2a, 2b, 3a & 3b**). In terms of histology, it is distinguished primarily by inflammatory cell infiltration and edema[1,2] (**Fig. 4**). On the fundic gland mucosa, mucosal swelling looks like soft, thick mucosa. In swollen areae gastricae (AG), the mucosa may appear uneven. Recognition of the AG pattern on the pyloric gland mucosa is often difficult in conventional endoscopy; the mucosa looks soft, somewhat thick, and shows some unevenness. In chromoendoscopy (contrast method), the AG pattern can be seen clearly (**Fig. 3c**), as is observed in the pattern on the fundic gland mucosa (**Fig. 2c**). This is very useful for assessment of mucosal swelling[1-3].

【Additional comments on areae gastricae】

The areae gastricae (AG) pattern can be seen clearly in chromoendoscopy (contrast method)[1-3]. In *H. pylori*-infected gastric mucosa, the AG is swollen and the surface appears taut, with narrow grooves between each area. In uninfected gastric mucosa, the mucosa does not look taut, the AG is not swollen, and the contours are jagged.

References

1) Kato T, Yagi N, Kamada T, et al : Diagnosis of *Helicobacter pylori* infection in gastric mucosa by endoscopic features : a multicenter prospective study. Dig Endosc 2013 ; 25 : 508-518
2) Nomura S, Terao S, Adachi K, et al : Endoscopic diagnosis of gastric mucosal activity and inflammation. Dig Endosc 2013 ; 25 : 136-146
3) Ida K, Kuroda M, Tsuboi H, et al. : [Comprehensive diagnosis of *H. pylori* infection using endoscopy.] Jpn Clin Gastroenterol 2001; 16: 1539-1546 (In Japanese)

6 Enlarged folds and tortuous folds

Yutaka Yamaji Yoshihiro Hirata

📖 Description ▶▶ Page 51

Fig. 1 Enlarged folds and tortuous folds (1)

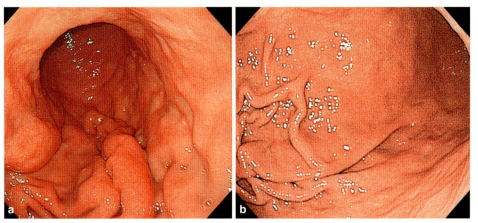

a: Before eradication   b: After eradication

a: Wide, curved folds can be seen, and the reddish color of the mucosa is very noticeable.
b: These findings are significantly reduced after *H. pylori* eradication.

Fig. 2 Enlarged folds and tortuous folds (2)

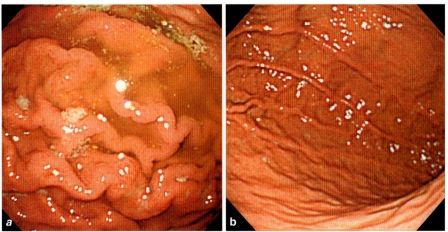

a: Before eradication   b: After eradication

a: As in Fig. 1, enlarged and tortuous folds are observed in the greater curvature of the corpus.
b: After *H. pylori* eradication, these findings decreased or disappeared.

• Equipment used (Pages 49–50)
  Endoscopes: GIF-H260 (Fig. 1), GIF-XQ240 (Fig. 2), GIF-Q240X (Fig. 3) (Olympus)
  Light source: EVIS LUCERA CLV-260SL (Olympus)

Fig. 3 Enlarged folds and tortuous folds (3)

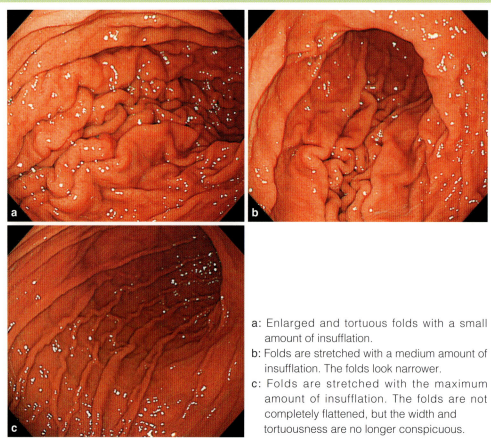

a: Enlarged and tortuous folds with a small amount of insufflation.
b: Folds are stretched with a medium amount of insufflation. The folds look narrower.
c: Folds are stretched with the maximum amount of insufflation. The folds are not completely flattened, but the width and tortuousness are no longer conspicuous.

Enlarged folds and tortuous folds

Description

In Shokaki Naishikyo Yogoshu (Gastrointestinal Endoscopy Terminology [in Japanese])[1] published by the Japan Gastroenterological Endoscopy Society, there is an entry for "giant fold, giant ruga," defining this as a wide, curved fold that resembles cerebral gyri. However, no clear criterion has been established yet.

The entry for "giant fold" in the glossary of terms of I to Cho (Stomach Intest)[2], states that although there is no clear definition, the term refers to a fold that is enlarged, in addition to exhibiting bending and tortuousness. The glossary goes on to state that the space between the folds is narrow and that a finding resembling cerebral gyri is exhibited when bending and tortuousness increase. Finally, it states that giant folds should be diagnosed when the following two conditions are observed: an X-ray shows that the folds have a width of more than 10 mm in double-contrast images with the gastric wall moderately stretched; and the folds still look enlarged in endoscopy even with sufficient insufflation.

In the rugal hyperplasia (fold enlargement) section of the Sydney System[3], an enlarged fold is defined as a fold that is not flattened or is only partially flattened by insufflation; a fold with a thickness of about 5 mm is minor, while one with a thickness of 5–10-mm thick is moderate, and anything over 10 mm is severe.

In endoscopic diagnosis, thickness and tortuousness should be obvious at a glance (**Figs. 1a & 2a**) and not disappear when the region is insufflated. However, the fold width varies considerably depending on the amount of insufflation (**Fig. 3**). After *H. pylori* eradication, the folds become noticeably thinner, even when the amount of insufflation is the same (**Figs. 1b & 2b**).

A cross-sectional study[4] and longitudinal study[5] have suggested that fold enlargement is a risk factor for undifferentiated gastric cancer. Problems remain, however. For example, the definition of fold enlargement is somewhat subjective and the natural history of fold enlargement has not yet been fully elucidated. Additional research in the future is expected to clarify these points.

References

1) Committee for terminology standardization of the Japan Gastroenterological Endoscopy Society (ed) : Shokaki Naishikyo Yogoshu [Gastrointestinal Endoscopy Terminology] (3rd edition). Tokyo: Igaku Shoin, 2011 (In Japanese)
2) Hamada T : [Giant folds, giant rugae.] I to Cho (Stomach Intest) 2012; 47 [Atlas: I to Cho Glossary of Terms 2012]: 690 (In Japanese)
3) Tytgat GN : The Sydney System : endoscopic division. Endoscopic appearances in gastritis/duodenitis. J Gastroenterol Hepatol 1991 ; 6 : 223-234
4) Nishibayashi H, Kanayama S, Kiyohara T, et al : *Helicobacter pylori*-induced enlarged-fold gastritis is associated with increased mutagenicity of gastric juice, increased oxidative DNA damage, and an increased risk of gastric carcinoma. J Gastroenterol Hepatol 2003 ; 18 : 1384-1391
5) Watanabe M, Kato J, Inoue I, et al: Development of gastric cancer in nonatrophic stomach with highly active inflammation identified by serum levels of pepsinogen and *Helicobacter pylori* antibody together with endoscopic rugal hyperplastic gastritis. Int J Cancer 2012; 131: 2632-2642

7 Nodularity

Tomoari Kamada

📖 Description ▶ Page 56

Fig. 1 Nodularity (1)

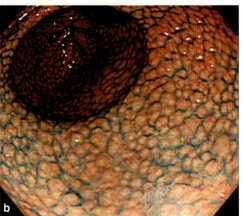

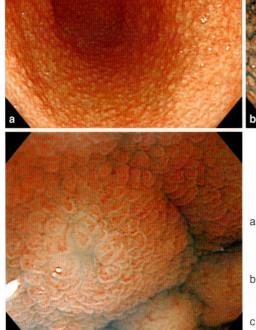

a: Uniform small granular elevations which shaped like cobblestones are heavily concentrated in the antrum (standard observation).
b: Indigo carmine spraying has made the elevations more prominent (dye-spraying chromoendoscopy).
c: A white depression can be seen in the center of each elevation (magnifying observation).

Fig. 2 Nodularity (2)

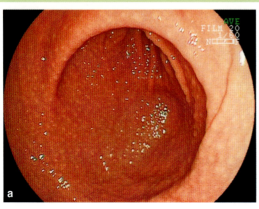

a: Small granular elevations can be seen in the antrum (standard observation).

2. Specific Discussions • 53

Fig. 2 Nodularity (2) cont'd

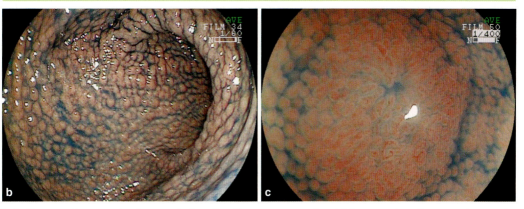

b: Indigo carmine spraying has made the elevations more prominent (dye-spraying chromoendoscopy).
c: A white depression can be seen in the center of each elevation (magnifying observation).

Fig. 3 Nodularity (3)

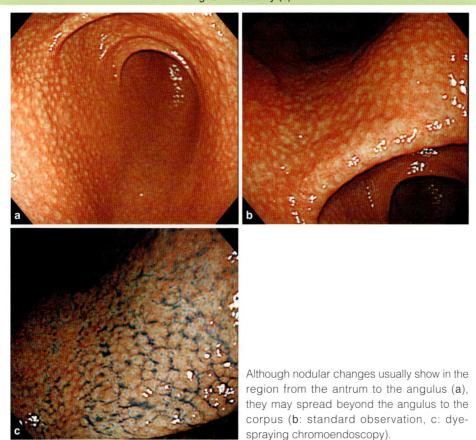

Although nodular changes usually show in the region from the antrum to the angulus (a), they may spread beyond the angulus to the corpus (b: standard observation, c: dye-spraying chromoendoscopy).

- Equipment used (Pages 52–55)
  Endoscopes: GIF-Q240 (Fig. 1), GIF-Q260 (Figs. 3 & 7), GIF-H260 (Fig. 4) (Olympus)
      Fujifilm (Figs. 2 & 5) (ultraslim model used in Fig. 5)

Fig. 4 Nodularity (4)

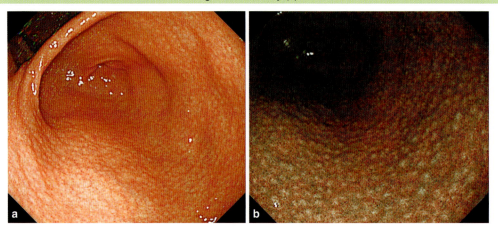

a: Small granular elevations can be seen in the antrum (WLI observation).
b: Under NBI observation, whitish granular elevations become clearly visible (NBI observation).

Fig. 5 Nodularity observed with an ultraslim endoscope

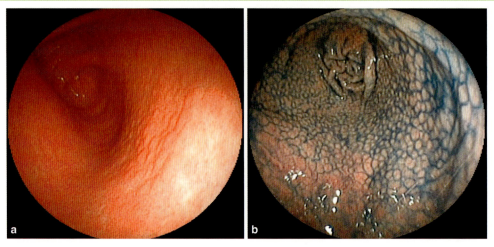

a: Standard observation   b: Dye-spraying chromoendoscopy
Nodular gastritis can be diagnosed even with an ultraslim endoscope.

Fig. 6 Biopsy specimen taken from nodularity (HE-stained)

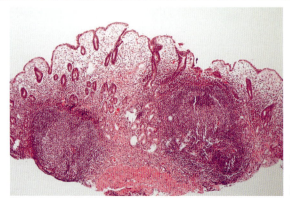

Image of typical specimen of nodularity. Large lymphoid follicles with germinal centers and severe inflammatory cell infiltration can be seen.

2. Specific Discussions 55

Fig. 7 Endoscopic images of nodularity before and after eradication

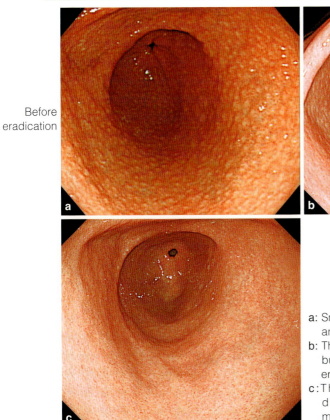

Before eradication

1 year after eradication

5 years after eradication

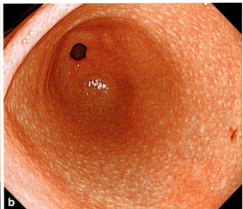

a: Small granular elevations can be seen in the antrum (before eradication).
b: The small granular elevations have flattened, but white dots still remain (1 year after eradication).
c: The small granular elevations have disappeared and become to atrophic mucosa (5 years after eradication).

Chapter 2 Endoscopic Findings of Gastritis

7. Nodularity

Nodularity

 Description

The condition in which uniform small granular elevations are concentrated on the gastric mucosa — like goosebumps — is called nodular gastric mucosa. These findings are often found in the region from the angulus to the antrum[1] (**Figs. 1–5**).

Traditionally, nodular gastric mucosa was regarded as a physiological phenomenon common in young women and was not believed to have much pathological significance. It was later discovered that nodular gastritis is an excessive immune response caused by a first-time *H. pylori* infection. This form of gastritis frequently occurs among *H. pylori*-positive children and young adults[2]. Researches have also reported cases of nodular gastritis with peptic ulcer and gastric cancer[3, 4]. As a result, it is now viewed as the important background of gastric cancer — especially undifferentiated gastric cancer — in young adult patients[5].

Endoscopic findings of nodular gastritis are distinguished by the appearance of nodules in the mucosa. White depressions can be seen in the centers of the nodular elevations (**Figs. 1c & 2c**). Pathologically, the essence of nodular gastritis is hyperplasia of lymphoid follicles (**Fig. 6**). Eradication causes these nodules to disappear over time.

A typical finding of nodular gastritis that suggests active *H. pylori* infection is the presence of clearly visible small granular elevations with a depression in the center of each elevation. When the elevations have flattened but white dots can still be seen (**Fig. 7**), nodular gastritis with *H. pylori* past-infection is the most likely explanation.

References

1) Takemoto T, Mizuno Y. : [Gastroscopic diagnosis of chronic gastritis and gastric biopsy.] Gastroenterol Endosc 1962; 4: 310–320 (In Japanese)
2) Konno M, Muraoka S. : [Characteristics of *Helicobacter pylori*-infected gastritis among children.] Helicobacter Res 1999; 3: 32–37 (In Japanese)
3) Miyamoto M, Haruma K, Yoshihara M, et al : Nodular gastritis in adults is caused by *Helicobacter pylori* infection. Dig Dis Sci 2003 ; 48 : 968-975
4) Miyamoto M, Haruma K, Yoshihara M, et al : Five cases of nodular gastritis and gastric cancer : a possible association between nodular gastritis and gastric cancer. Dig Liver Dis 2003 ; 34 : 819-820
5) Kamada T, Haruma K, Sugiu K, et al : Case of early gastric cancer with nodular gastritis. Dig Endosc 2004 ; 16 : 39-43

2. Specific Discussions • 57

8 Foveolar-hyperplastic polyp

Masanori Ito

📖 Description ▶▶ Page 59

Fig. 1 Foveolar-hyperplastic polyp generated in the cardia

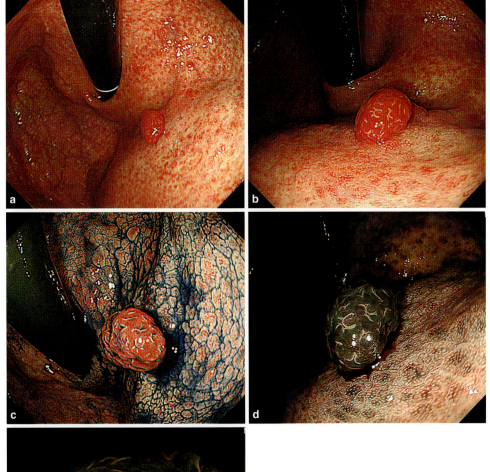

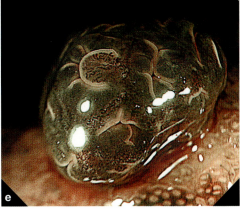

Female in her 70s. A reddish Yamada's Type II polyp is present on atrophic mucosa infected by *H. pylori*. A large mucosal pattern and microvascular expansion with regularity maintained are also present.
a: WLI image. b: Close-up image.
c: Indigo carmine sprayed image.
d: NBI image.
e: Magnifying image [d, e: Structure Enhancement — A7, Color Enhancement — 1].

58 ● Chapter 2 Endoscopic Findings of Gastritis

Fig. 2 Foveolar-hyperplastic polyp reduced by eradication therapy

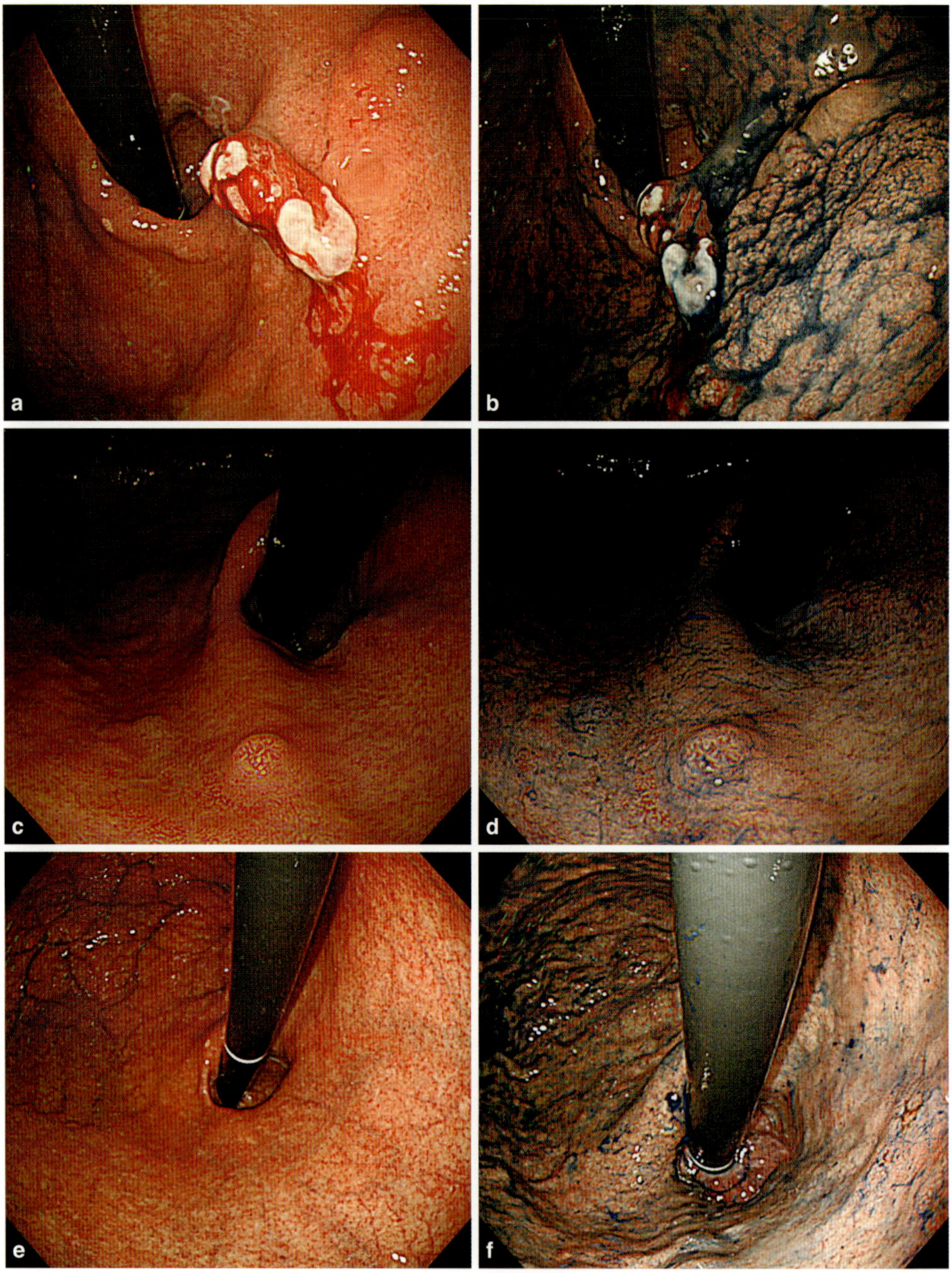

Before eradication

2 years after eradication

5 years after eradication

Male in his 70s. A hyperplastic polyp accompanied by hemorrhage and white coat attachment was recognized in the gastric cardia. After *H. pylori* eradication, the polyp gradually reduced in size over a 5 year period.
Top row (**a**, **b**): Before eradication. Middle row (**c**, **d**): 2 years after eradication. Bottom row: 5 years after eradication.
WLI images on the left (**a**, **c**, **e**) and indigo carmine sprayed images on the right (**b**, **d**, **f**).

● Equipment used (Pages 57–58)
  Endoscope: GIF–H260 (Olympus)
  Light source: EVIS LUCERA CLV–260SL (Olympus)

Foveolar-hyperplastic polyp

Description

Due to its vascular density, a foveolar-hyperplastic polyp looks redder than normal mucosa (**Fig. 1**) and is often accompanied by mucus and a white coating[1]. Under NBI observation, mucosal patterns look larger and microvascular expansion is visible. The shape of these patterns is uniform and vascular regularity is maintained[2]. Foveolar -hyperplastic polyps can be found any region from the cardia to the pylorus. They are found in gastric mucosa with *H. pylori* infection and often appear based on atrophic background[3].

Histologically speaking, hyperplastic change in the foveolar epithelium is the primary finding. Ducts exhibit elongation, branching, and expansion. This is sometimes accompanied by mild nuclear enlargement caused by regenerative changes[4].

Under normal circumstances without treatment, foveolar-hyperplastic polyps usually remain as they are or increase in size. Virtually none of them disappear. However, once *H. pylori* eradication has been performed, they often disappear or become smaller[5] (**Fig. 2**). While occurrence rates are low, foveolar-hyperplastic polyps may coexist with carcinoma or they could bleed, resulting in iron-deficiency anemia. To avoid this, endoscopic resection is recommended.

References

1) Akamatsu T, Shimodaira K, Matsuzawa K, et al. : [Differential diagnosis of gastric elevated lesions in white light imaging.] I to Cho (Stomach Intest) 2012; 47: 1200–1208 (In Japanese)
2) Yamashina T, Uedo N, Ishihara R, et al. : [Classification and differentiation of gastric polyps — characteristics in NBI magnifying observation.] I to Cho (Stomach Intest) 2012; 47: 1209–1215 (In Japanese)
3) Haruma K, Yoshihara M, Sumii K, et al : Gastric acid secretion, serum pepsinogen I, and serum gastrin in Japanese with gastric hyperplastic polyps or polypoid-type early gastric carcinoma. Scand J Gastroenterol 1993 ; 28 : 633-637
4) Yao T, Mitomi H, Hidaka Y, et al. : [Pathological classification, differential diagnosis and clinical significance of gastric polyps.] I to Cho (Stomach Intest) 2012; 47: 1192–1199 (In Japanese)
5) Okusa T, Horiuchi H, Arakawa H, et al. : [Natural history of gastric polyps and malignant potential — foveolar-hyperplastic polyps.] I to Cho (Stomach Intest) 2012; 47: 1216–1226 (In Japanese)

9 Xanthoma

Shinji Kitamura

📖 Description ▶ Page 62

Fig. 1 Lesions in the antrum

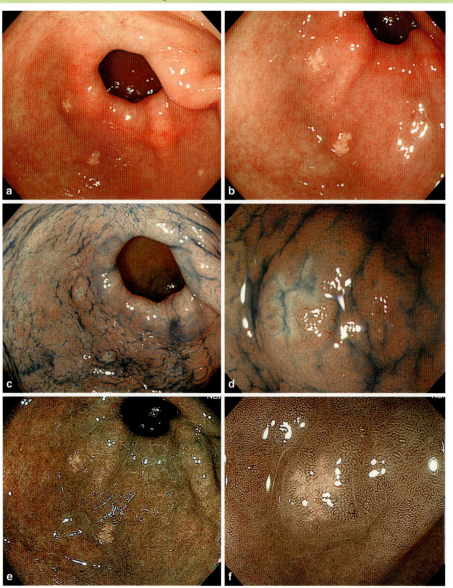

a, b: Xanthoma in the antrum. Multiple small star-like yellowish-white spots with well-defined margins can be seen in the vicinity of the pyloric ring.

c, d: Indigo carmine sprayed images. The lesion is flat and its surface shows a fine granular structure.

e, f: NBI images. The lesion appears whitish with distinct margins. The fine granularity of the surface structure is clear. [Structure Enhancement: B8; Color Enhancement: 1]

- Equipment used (Pages 60–61)
  Endoscopes: GIF-H260Z (Fig. 1), GIF-HQ290 (Fig. 2) (Olympus)
  Light sources: EVIS LUCERA CLV-260SL, (Fig. 1), EVIS LUCERA CLV-290SL (Fig. 2) (Olympus)

Fig. 2 Lesions in the corpus

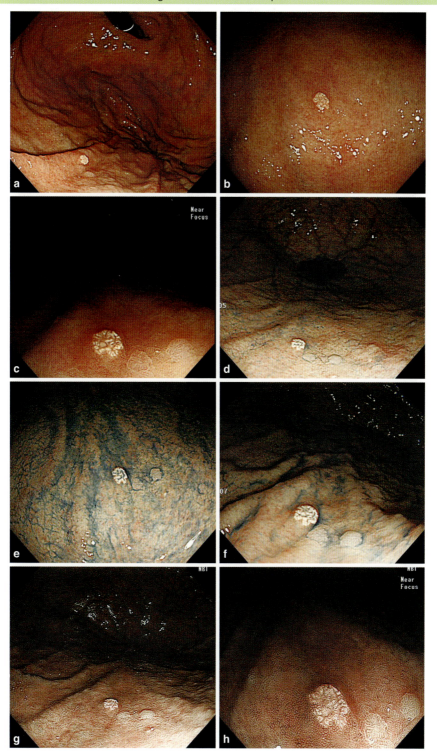

a, b, c: Xanthoma in the corpus. Yellowish-white, oval, slightly elevated lesions with distinct margins can be seen. The surface structure features fine granularity.

d, e, f: Indigo carmine sprayed images. These are lightly elevated lesions with fine granularity and distinct margins. Groove-like pools of indigo carmine can be seen between the granules.

g, h: NBI images. The lesions are bright and whitish with distinct margins. They exhibit a fine granular surface pattern. [Structure Enhancement: B8; Color Enhancement: 1]

Fig. 3 Histological finding (HE)

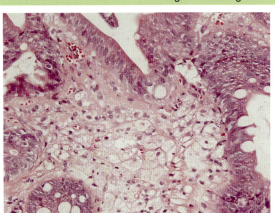

Bright round vacuolated cells (xanthoma cells) can be seen in the superficial layer of the lamina propria mucosae.

Xanthoma

📖 Description

Xanthoma or xanthelasma is a flat or slightly elevated lesion that ranges in color from whitish to yellowish and has a surface structure that exhibits fine granularity (**Figs. 1 & 2**). It is typically observed in gastritis currently or previously associated with a *H. pylori* infection. In the histological image (**Fig. 3**), round vacuolated cells (xanthoma cells) can be seen in the superficial layer of the lamina propria mucosae. This is considered to be an aggregation of histiocytes that have phagocytosed lipid. Xanthoma remains even after *H. pylori* eradication.

References

1) Kimura K, Hiramoto T and Buncher CR : Gastric xanthelasma. Arch Pathol 1969 ; 87 : 110-117
2) Kaiserling E, Heinle H, Itabe H, et al : Lipid islands in human gastric mucosa : morphological and immunohistochemical findings. Gastroenterology 1996 ; 110 : 369-374
3) Hori S, Tsutsumi Y : *Helicobacter pylori* infection in gastric xanthomas : immunohistochemical analysis of 145 lesions. Pathol Int 1966 ; 46 : 589-593
4) Sekikawa A, Fukui H, Maruo T, et al : Gastric xanthelasma may be a warning sign for the presence of early gastric cancer. J Gastroenterol Hepatol 2014 ; 29 : 951-956

2. Specific Discussions

10 Depressive erosion

Yoshihiro Hirata

📖 Description ▶▶ Page 65

Fig. 1 Small depressive erosion in the lesser curvature of the pyloric antrum

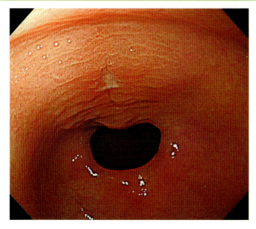

Depressive erosion that emerged on *H. pylori*-negative gastric mucosa.

Fig. 2 Multiple depressive erosions around the pyloric ring

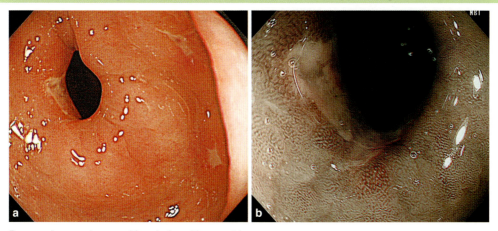

Depressive erosions on *H. pylori*-positive gastric mucosa.
a: WLI observation. b: NBI [Structure Enhancement — B8, Color Enhancement — 1].

• Equipment used (Pages 63–65)
 Endoscopes: GIF-Q240X (Figs. 1, 4c, 5b), GIF-XQ240 (Figs. 4a, 4b), GIF-H260 (Fig. 5a),
    GIF-H260Z (Figs. 2, 3) (Olympus)
Light source: EVIS LUCERA CLV-260SL (Olympus)

Fig. 3　Depressive erosion on the posterior wall of the antrum

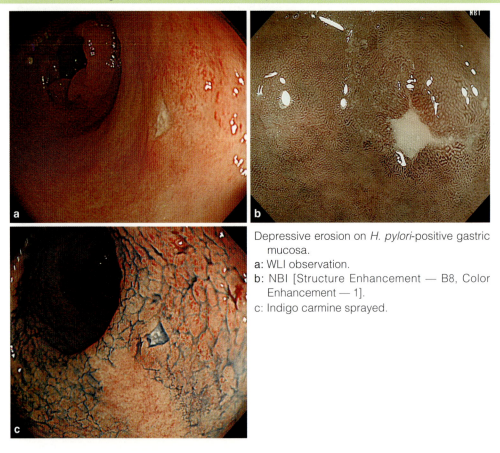

Depressive erosion on *H. pylori*-positive gastric mucosa.
a: WLI observation.
b: NBI [Structure Enhancement — B8, Color Enhancement — 1].
c: Indigo carmine sprayed.

Fig. 4　Depressive erosion of rheumatoid arthritis (RA) patient taking NSAID medication

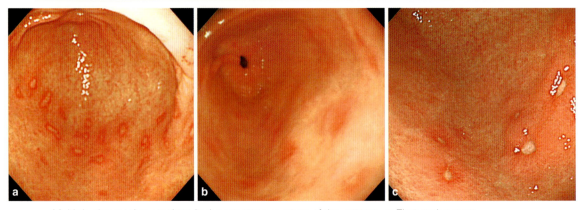

Multiple depressive erosions in the greater curvature of the antrum. a: First endoscopy.
b: After cessation of NSAID medication. c: After resumption of NSAID medication.

Fig. 5 Depressive erosion in the middle corpus

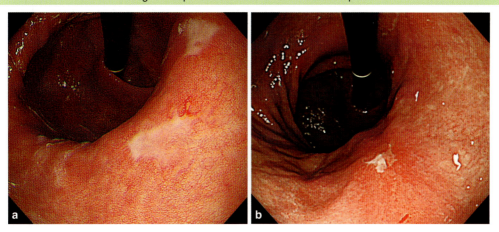

Shallow depressive erosion seen in RA patient taking steroid/immunosuppressant medication. Immunostaining of pathological tissue showed cytomegalovirus (CMV) positive.
a: Before treatment. b: After antiviral treatment.

Depressive erosion

Description

Erosion is a condition in which the epithelium is deficient and continuity is lost. Tissue loss depresses the erosion site, while the epithelial cells around the deficient part of the epithelium are flat. This is called depressive erosion (**Figs. 1–3**). Histologically, depressive erosion is an epithelial cell deficiency in the mucosal layer that penetrates no deeper than the lamina muscularis mucosae (UI-I when expressed in terms of the depth of the gastric ulcer).

The causes of erosion can be acid secretion, chemical/physical stimuli, drugs (**Fig. 4**), *H. pylori* infection, *H. pylori* eradication (recovery of acid secretion accompanied by it), and viral infection (**Fig. 5**), etc. Erosion often occurs in multiple locations[1)–5)]. When solitary depressive erosion is observed, it is important to differentiate it from early carcinoma.

References

1) Kato T, Yagi N, Kamada T, et al ; Study Group for Establishing Endoscopic Diagnosis of Chronic Gastritis : Diagnosis of *Helicobacter pylori* infection in gastric mucosa by endoscopic features : a multicenter prospective study. Dig Endosc 2013 ; 25 : 508-518
2) Toljamo KT, Niemelä SE, Karvonen AL, et al : Evolution of gastritis in patients with gastric erosions. Scand J Gastroenterol 2005 ; 40 : 1275-1283
3) Kodama T, Fukuda S, Takino T, et al : Gastroduodenal cytomegalovirus infection after renal transplantation. Fiberscopic observations. Endoscopy 1985 ; 17 : 157-158
4) Watanabe K, Hoshiya S, Tokunaga K, et al. : [The clinical importance of mucosal lesions in the upper gastrointestinal tract after the eradication of *Helicobacter pylori* infection.] Gastroenterol Endosc 2000; 42: 807–815 (In Japanese)
5) Kanno K. : [NSAID and gastrointestinal disorders.] J JSGE 2009; 106: 321-326 (In Japanese)

11 Regular arrangement of collecting venules (RAC)

Kazuyoshi Yagi

📖 Description ▶▶ Page 67

Fig. 1 RAC images in the lower corpus

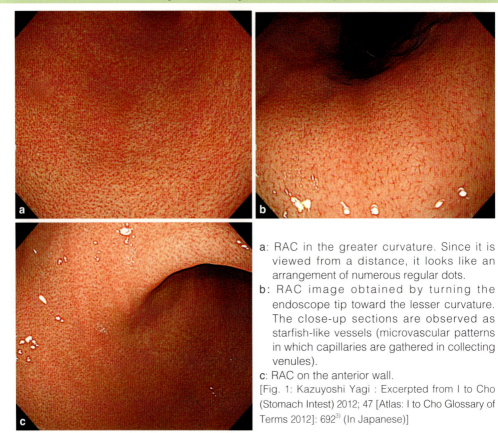

a: RAC in the greater curvature. Since it is viewed from a distance, it looks like an arrangement of numerous regular dots.
b: RAC image obtained by turning the endoscope tip toward the lesser curvature. The close-up sections are observed as starfish-like vessels (microvascular patterns in which capillaries are gathered in collecting venules).
c: RAC on the anterior wall.
[Fig. 1: Kazuyoshi Yagi : Excerpted from I to Cho (Stomach Intest) 2012; 47 [Atlas: I to Cho Glossary of Terms 2012]: 692[3)] (In Japanese)]

Fig. 2 RAC images in the region from the angulus to the lesser curvature of the antrum

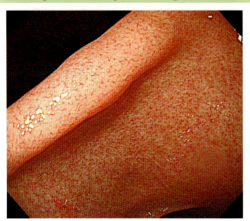

Viewed up close, the angulus looks like a collection of as starfish-like vessels. The antrum looks like an arrangement of numerous regular dots since it was viewed from distance.
[Fig. 2: Kazuyoshi Yagi : Excerpted from I to Cho (Stomach Intest) 2012; 47 [Atlas: I to Cho Glossary of Terms 2012]: 692[3)] (In Japanese)]

RAC

📖 Description

RAC (regular arrangement of collecting venules) is an endoscopically observed condition in which collecting venues are arranged regularly in the corpus. From a distance, it looks like numerous dots (**Fig. 1a**). From up close, it looks like a regular arrangement of starfish-like patterns (**Fig. 1b**). When RAC is observed throughout the corpus, the stomach is considered to be RAC-positive, in which case it is diagnosed as normal and not infected with *H. pylori*[1), 2)]. When a stomach is judged RAC-positive and diagnosed as normal with no *H. pylori* infection, the diagnostic accuracy rate is 95%[1), 2)].

In antrum-dominant gastritis where there is little inflammation in the upper corpus, RAC-resemblant (pseudo-RAC) endoscopic images are sometimes observed in the upper corpus of an *H. pylori*-infected stomach with a small atrophic area — a duodenal ulcer, for example. Even in cases like this, RAC images often disappear in the lower corpus and angulus. Consequently, it is recommended to examine the lower corpus or angulus (**Fig. 1c**) when assessing whether or not the stomach is RAC positive. In a typical *H.pylori*-uninfected stomach, RAC is also observed in the region from the angulus to the lesser curvature of the antrum (**Fig. 2**)[1)].

References

1) Yagi K, Nakamura A, Sekine A, et al. : [Endoscopic features of the normal gastric mucosa without *Helicobacter pylori* infection.] Gastroenterol Endosc 2000; 42: 1977–1987 (In Japanese)
2) Yagi K, Nakamura A and Sekine A : Characteristic endoscopic and magnified endoscopic findings in the normal stomach without *Helicobacter pylori* infection. J Gastroenterol Hepatol 2002 ; 17 : 39-45
3) Yagi K: [RAC.] I to Cho (Stomach Intest) 2012; 47 [Atlas: I to Cho Glossary of Terms 2012]: 692 (In Japanese)

• Equipment used (Page 66)
  Endoscopes: GIF-H260Z (Olympus)
  Light source: EVIS LUCERA CLV-260SL (Olympus)

12 Fundic gland polyp

Kazuhiko Inoue

📖 Description ▸▸ Page 70

Fig. 1 Fundic gland polyp (1)

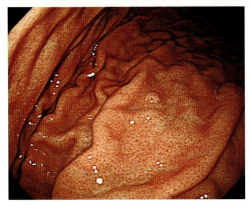

Small Yamada's Type II elevations with the same color tone as the surrounding mucosa can be seen in the fundic gland region of normal gastric mucosa with no *H. pylori* infection.

Fig. 2 Fundic gland polyp (2)

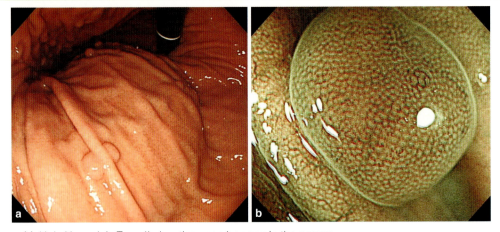

a: Multiple Yamada's Type II elevations can be seen in the corpus.
b: In NBI magnifying observation, round-to-oval crypt openings can be seen.

Fig. 3 Fundic gland polyp (3)

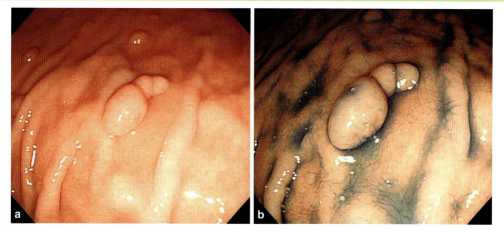

a: A slightly large polyp with Yamada's Type III morphology.
b: The surface looks smooth even when sprayed with dye.

Fig. 4 Fundic gland polyp (4)

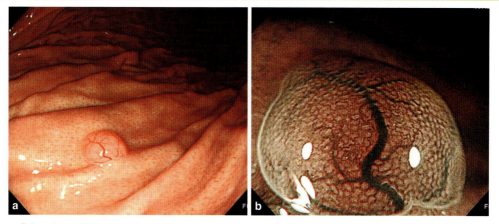

a: Dilated vessels can be seen on the surface of the polyp.
b: In NBI magnifying observation, these vessels are highlighted with cyan.

Fig. 5 Histological finding

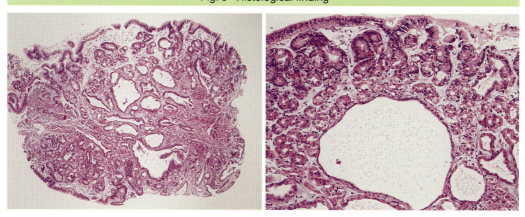

The specimen features hyperplasia of fundic gland tissue and dilated cystic glands.

Fig. 6 Fundic gland polyposis seen in familial adenomatous polyposis (FAP)

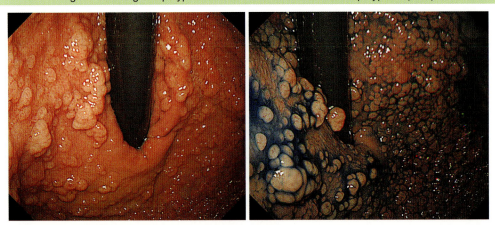

Fundic gland polyp

Description

Fundic gland polyps are generated in the fundic gland region (corpus and fornix). Most of them are small and smooth, measuring a few millimeters across, and exhibit Yamada's Type II. Their color tone usually matches that of the surrounding mucosa (**Figs. 1 & 2**). Polyps measuring more than 5 millimeters tend to exhibit Yamada's Type III (**Fig. 3**). In NBI observation, crypt openings can be seen. The shape of these openings ranges from round to oval (**Fig. 2b**), and they are sometimes accompanied by dilated vessels with a cyan color tone (**Fig. 4b**).

Histologically (**Fig. 5**), a fundic gland polyp is an elevated lesion that features hyperplasia of fundic gland tissue and dilated cystic glands[1].

Fundic gland polyps are usually found in normal gastric mucosa free from *H. pylori* infection, inflammation, or atrophy. The risk of gastric cancer is very low[2]–[4]. Long-term proton pump inhibitor administration may generate new fundic gland polyps and increase the size of existing polyps[5]. They may also appear after successful *H. pylori* eradication.

Fundic gland polyposis accompanied by familial adenomatous polyposis (FAP) can be the basis of cancer (**Fig. 6**)

References

1) Kamada T, Inoue K, Aoki T, et al. : [Natural history of gastric polyps and malignant potential — fundic gland polyps.] I to Cho (Stomach Intest) 2012; 47: 1227–1234 (In Japanese)
2) Haruma K, Sumii K, Morikawa A, et al. : [Investigation into the background gastric mucosa of hyperplastic fundic gland polyps.] J JSGE 1989; 86: 851–857 (In Japanese)
3) Uemura N, Mukai S, Yamaguchi S, et al. : [Clinical investigation into the background gastric mucosa in fundic gland polyp cases — especially in comparison with gastric cancer cases.] Gastroenterol Endosc 1993; 35: 2663–2671 (In Japanese)
4) Inoue K, Fujisawa T and Haruma K : Assessment of degree of health of the stomach by concomitant measurement of serum pepsinogen and serum *Helicobacter pylori* antibodies. Int J Biol Markers 2010 ; 25 : 207–212
5) Hongo M and Fujimoto K ; Gastric Polyps Study Group : Incidence and risk factor of fundic gland polyp and hyperplastic polyp in long-term proton pump inhibitor therapy : a prospective study in Japan. J Gastroenterol 2010 ; 45 : 618–624

13 Red streak

Susumu Ohwada   Masayuki Inui
Naondo Sohara   Yoshikatsu Inui

📖 Description ▶▶ Page 74

Fig. 1   Red streak (1)

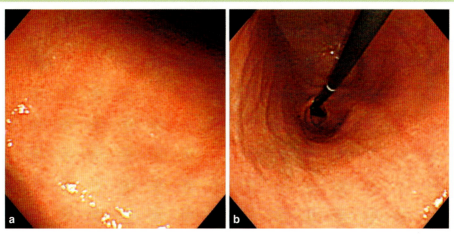

Female, 77 years old. Symptoms: none.
a: Numerous pale red streaks can be seen in the lesser curvature of the corpus.
b: RAC (regular arrangement of collecting venules) can be seen in the background mucosa of the lesser curvature of the corpus. Numerous pale red streaks can also be seen.

Fig. 2   Red streak (2)

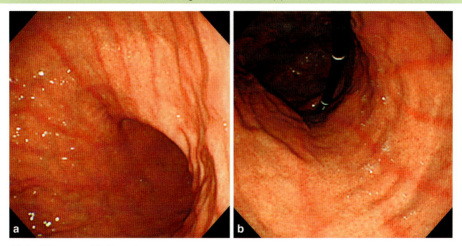

Male, 64 years old. Symptoms: none.
a: Numerous bright red streaks can be seen in the region from the lesser curvature to the greater curvature of the corpus.
b: RAC can be seen in the background mucosa of the lesser curvature of the corpus. Numerous pale red streaks can also be seen.

Fig. 3 Red streak (3)

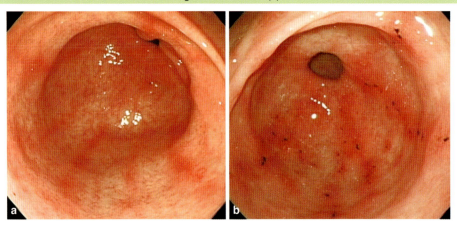

a: Male, 57 years old. Symptoms: minor abdominal pain. Numerous partially swollen red streaks can be seen in the region from the lesser curvature to the greater curvature of the antrum. He complained of minor abdominal pain.

b: Male, 69 years old. Symptoms: minor abdominal pain. As in the case shown in Fig. 3a, numerous partially swollen red streaks can be seen in the greater curvature of the antrum. Attachment of hematin is also observed. This patient also complained of minor abdominal pain.

Fig. 4 Red streak (4)

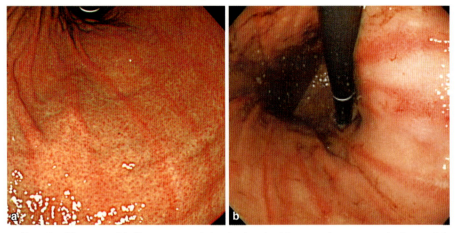

a: Female, 70 years old. Symptoms: abdominal pain. The gastric mucosa looks as if it were imaged with the Color and Structure Enhancement levels increased. Numerous swollen red streaks can be seen in the lesser curvature of the antrum. As RAC shows hyperemia, redness is emphasized. She complained of strong abdominal pain.

b: Female, 57 years old. Symptoms: none. Numerous bright red streaks can be seen in the entirety of the stomach from the lesser curvature to the greater curvature of the corpus. The red streaks on the lesser curvature side are swollen. Some of the crests have erosion, and attachment of hematin is also recognized on the red streaks on the greater curvature side. However, this patient did not complain of abdominal pain.

- Equipment used (Pages 71–73)
  Endoscopes: GIF-XP260N (Fig. 1), GIF-XP260NS (Fig. 2), GIF-H260 (Figs. 3–5) (Olympus)
  Light sources: EVIS LUCERA SPECTRUM CLV-260NBI (Fig. 1), EVIS LUCERA ELITE CLV-290 (Fig. 2),
  EVIS LUCERA SPECTRUM CLV-260SL (Figs. 3–5) (Olympus)

Fig. 5 Red streak (5)

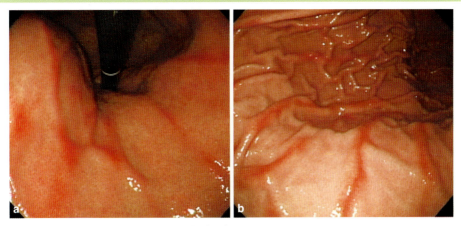

Male, 16 years old. Symptoms: abdominal pain.
a: RAC can be seen on the mucosa in the lesser curvature of the corpus. Three partially swollen medium-degree bright red streaks are also visible.
b: Four extremely bright red streaks are visible in the greater curvature of the corpus. Their crests also have erosion. The patient complained of severe abdominal pain.

Red streak

Description

Red streaks are strips in red that run longitudinally along the long axis of the stomach. A few red streaks run almost parallely[1]. They are usually seen on the crests of the folds. Their original German name, Kammrötung[2] means "comb-like redness". The Japan Gastroenterological Endoscopy Society recently updates its terminology, abandoning the term "comb-like redness" and changing it to "red streak"[1]. Redness (erythema or hyperemia) is distinguishable because it looks redder than the surrounding mucosa. When viewed from up close, it is aggregation of numerous very small red dots, so it is also called fine pink speckling. Sometimes, depressions accompanied by strip-like or groove-like gaps with a white coating are seen in the center of the band-like redness. Attachment of hematin is also sometimes seen. Red streaks may also be localized in the lesser curvature of the corpus and the greater curvature of the antrum, as well as extending from the greater curvature of the corpus to the entire stomach (**Figs. 1 & 2**). The colors of red streaks range from pink to bright red, and their severity is classified as minor, moderate, and severe[3]. A red streak is redness that appears on the surface that comes in contact with gastric juice when the stomach is contracted. Under magnifying endoscopy, it becomes apparent that the redness is caused by congestion of capillary networks in the superficial layer of the mucosa.

Red streaks are usually seen in mucosa that is not infected by *H. pylori* and where gastritis is not present (all cases shown in Figs. 1–5 are *H. pylori*-uninfected). They may also be seen after *H. pylori* eradication[4]. Red streaks are found frequently in young females and tend to decrease in frequency with age. Generally, the more severe the red streaks, the higher the frequency of abdominal pain[5] (**Figs. 3–5**).

The origin of red streaks is not clear; it is considered that functional ones are possible. Even pathological findings are not specific. In cases where groove-like depressions can be seen in the center, acute inflammation — such as edema or cell infiltration— is observed endoscopically. Red streaks were regarded as a finding for superficial gastritis, but this has since come into question from a pathological perpective[3].

Findings of red streaks are also seen in resected stomachs. In this case, the streaks are believed to be the result of inflammation caused by bile reflux.

References

1) Committee for terminology standardization of the Japan Gastroenterological Endoscopy Society (ed) : [Terminology regarding endoscopic findings — detailed description.] Shokaki Naishikyo Yogoshu ([Gastrointestinal Endoscopy Terminology]) (3rd edition). Tokyo: Igaku Shoin, 2011, 90–91 (In Japanese)
2) Henning N. Krankheiten des Magens. In: Lehrbuch der Verdauungskrankheiten. 1949, p.118, Georg Thieme, Stuttgart
3) Okazaki Y, Takeo S : [Red streaks (Kammrötung).] I to Cho (Stomach Intest) 2012; 47 [Atlas: I to Cho Glossary of Terms 2012]: 691 (In Japanese)
4) Uemura N : [*H. pylori* infection and endoscopic images.] Gastroenterol Endosc 2005; 47: 2139–2145 (In Japanese)
5) Iwai C, Kitahora T, Ito H, et al : [Investigation into Kammrötung from the viewpoint of active oxygen amount generated in gastric mucosal tissue.] Gastroenterol Endosc 1993; 35: 1711(In Japanese)

14 Raised erosion

Takashi Kawai

📖 Description ▶▶ Page 76

Fig. 1 *H. pylori*-negative case

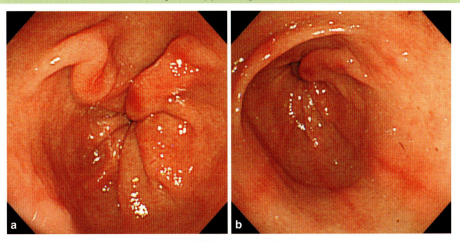

Female in her 50s. *H. pylori*-negative (UBT value: 0.3‰).
a: Raised erosion can be seen along the lesser curvature and posterior wall of the pylorus. There is a white depression in the center of the erosion.
b: There are red streaks on the greater curvature side.

Fig. 2 *H. pylori*-positive case

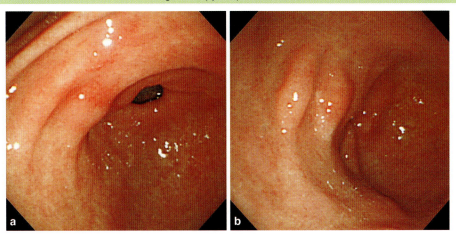

a: Male in his 60s. *H. pylori*-positive (UBT value: 3.2‰). A raised edematous erosion with a moderate slope and accompanied by redness covers the lesser curvature of the pylorus.
b: Male in his 70s. *H. pylori*-positive (UBT value: 41.9‰). A raised edematous erosion that extends in the direction of the short axis is recognized in the lesser curvature of the pyloric antrum.

Raised erosion

Description

A raised erosion is what Japanese physicians call an "octopus-sucker" erosion (verrucous gastritis) and is also entered in the Updated Sydney System[1]. It can manifest as polyps, clubs, or a string of beads. Typically, there are multiple occurrences but sometimes there may be just a single occurrence. A white depression is frequently present in in the center of the erosion. Although raised erosions tend to occur in the antrum, they are also found in the corpus. As for *H. pylori* infection, the study by Kato et al. found little correlation between the presence of raised erosions and *H. pylori* infection[2].

In terms of endoscopic morphological characteristics and the presence/absence of *H. pylori* infection, *H. pylori*-negative raised erosions (**Fig. 1**) are often recognized as verrucous erosions on the lesser curvature side and are accompanied by red streaks (long-axis direction). In most cases, there are no edematous changes in the mucosa. Similarly, with *H. pylori*-positive erosion (**Fig. 2**), erosion is likewise recognized on the lesser curvature side. However, in this case, raising occurs on the anterior and posterior walls (short-axis direction) and is rarely accompanied by red streaks. It is also often accompanied by edematous changes to the entire mucosa.

References

1) Dixon MF, Genta RM, Yardley JH, et al : Classification and grading of gastritis. The updated Sydney System. International Workshop on the Histopathology of Gastritis, Houston 1994. Am J Surg Pathol 1996 ; 20 : 1161-1181
2) Kato T, Yagi N, Kamada T, et al ; Study Group for Establishing Endoscopic Diagnosis of Chronic Gastritis : Diagnosis of *Helicobacter pylori* infection in gastric mucosa by endoscopic features : a multicenter prospective study. Dig Endosc 2013 ; 25 : 508-518

- Equipment used (Page 75)
  Endoscope: GIF-XP260NS (Olympus)
  Light source: EVIS LUCERA SPECTRUM CLV-260SL (Olympus)

15 Hematin

Hironori Masuyama

📖 Description ▶▶ Page 78

Fig. 1 Hematin in the antrum seen in an *H. pylori*-uninfected stomach

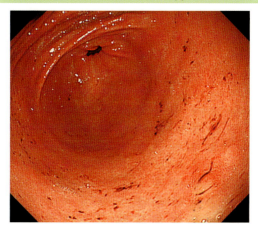

Fig. 2 Hematin seen after *H. pylori* eradication

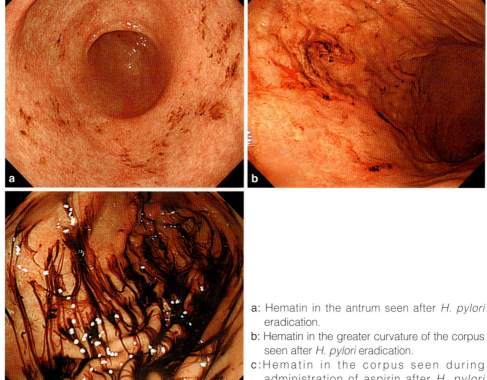

a: Hematin in the antrum seen after *H. pylori* eradication.
b: Hematin in the greater curvature of the corpus seen after *H. pylori* eradication.
c: Hematin in the corpus seen during administration of aspirin after *H. pylori* eradication.

Hematin

Description

Hematin attached on the gastric mucosa is from old blood components and is in most cases believed to be caused by gastric mucosal bleeding.

It is well known that hematin attachment is often seen on the gastric mucosa of *H. pylori*-uninfected patients (**Fig. 1**); however, it has been recently reported that it is also produced by changes to the gastric mucosa after *H. pylori* eradication (**Figs. 2a & 2b**)[1), 2)]. It is also seen in *H. pylori*-infected patients, as well as in patients who have been taking NSAIDs, aspirin, and other antithrombotic agents. In 100 *H. pylori*-uninfected cases experienced by this author, the occurrence frequency of hematin attachment was 15.0%.

Various studies have reported that the occurrence frequency of hematin after *H. pylori* eradication ranges from 4.8%[1)] to 17.5%[2)] and that most lesions are generated immediately after eradication. While hematin can be generated anywhere in the stomach, reports suggest that it is most frequently generated in the lower stomach (angulus and antrum)[2)].

It is believed that the recovery of gastric acid secretion[3)] after eradication is what causes the occurrence of hematin. In *H. pylori*-uninfected cases, maintenance of gastric acid secretion is thought to be a cause. Although attachment of hematin is not usually a concern, it can become a problem when patients are taking antithrombotic agents (**Fig. 2c**), so caution should be exercised.

References

1) Ono S, Kato M, Suzuki M, et al : [Differentiation between benign and malignant gastric erosion and redness after *H. pylori* eradication.] Gastroenterol Endosc 2011; 23: 1761–1766 (In Japanese)
2) Matsuhisa T, Kusakabe S, Maeda S, et al : [Observation of esophageal, gastric, and duodenal lesions after *Helicobacter pylori* eradication.] Ther Res 2001; 22: 1872–1874 (In Japanese)
3) El-Omar EM, Oien K, El-Nujumi A, et al : *Helicobacter pylori* infection and chronic gastric acid hyposecretion. Gastroenterology 1997 ; 113 : 15-24

• Equipment used (Page 77)
　Endoscopes: GIF-PQ260 (Figs. 1 & 2a), GIF-H260 (Figs. 2b & 2c) (Olympus)
　Light source: EVIS LUCERA SPECTRUM CLV-260SL (Olympus)

16 Corpus erosion

Shigemi Nakajima

📖 Description ▶▶Page 82

Fig. 1 Corpus erosion (crest erosion) in an *H. pylori*-uninfected stomach

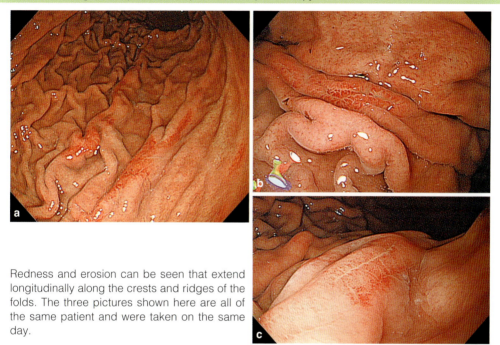

Redness and erosion can be seen that extend longitudinally along the crests and ridges of the folds. The three pictures shown here are all of the same patient and were taken on the same day.

Fig. 2 Corpus erosion (raised erosion) after *H. pylori* eradication

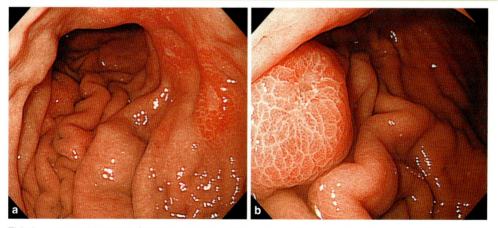

This is a case with gastric/duodenal ulcers. About six months after *H. pylori* eradication, multiple new raised erosions have become apparent in the stomach. The erosion does not show any signs of malignancy. New erosions have emerged in the corpus. Endoscopically, the background gastric mucosa of the corpus no longer exhibits diffuse redness and the mucosal surface has become smooth and glossy, indicating that the eradication treatment has been successful.

80 • Chapter 2 Endoscopic Findings of Gastritis

Fig. 3 A case with chronic gastritis 5 months after *H. pylori* eradication (raised erosion, possibly a type of crest erosion?)

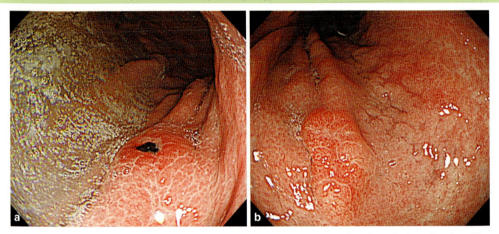

In this case, multiple new raised erosions can be seen five months after *H. pylori* eradication. The erosions can be seen on both the crests and ridges, as well as their extension lines. Some of the erosions have hematin attached, which is believed to have bled from the erosions. The fact that the erosions emerged after the eradication, while the diffuse redness in the background gastric mucosa has disappeared, the mucosal surface has become smoother, and small patches of map-like redness are visible, indicates that the eradication treatment has been successful.

Fig. 4 Corpus linear erosion in an *H. pylori*-positive patient

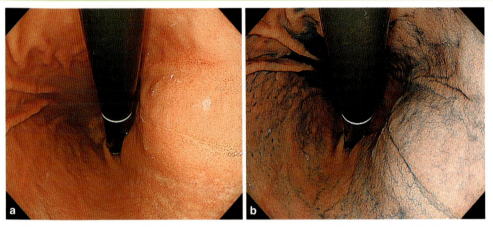

In this case, linear or longitudinal erosions have appeared on the opposite side (the lesser curvature side) of the greater curvature of the corpus — as if mirroring the folds. An indigo-carmine sprayed image is shown in figure 4b. Because this patient had been prescribed a proton pump inhibitor, the mucosal surface image looks at first glance as if it were *H. pylori* negative; however, it was positive.

• Equipment used (Pages 79–81)
  Endoscopes: GIF-Q240 (Figs. 1 & 2); GIF-H260Z (Figs. 3–5) (Olympus)
  Light source: EVIS LUCERA SPECTRUM CLV-260SL (Olympus)

Fig. 5 Longitudinal erosion in the lesser curvature of the corpus of an *H. pylori*-positive patient

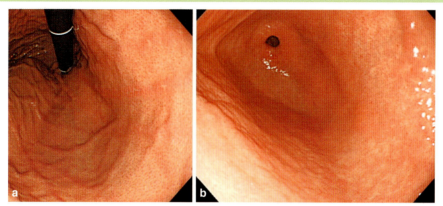

Multiple small and irregularly shaped erosions arranged lengthwise can be seen along the lesser curvature of the corpus (**a**). They look like long red streaks. Based on findings of the background mucosa in the corpus, this case was initially thought to be *H. pylori*-negative. However, the coarseness of the mucosal texture in the antrum (**b**), and a culture test made it clear that it was *H. pylori*-positive. While longitudinal redness in the lesser curvature of the corpus is a finding typical of *H. pylori*-negative stomachs, the fact that in this case the longitudinal redness was accompanied by coarse mucosal texture in the antrum indicates that the endoscopic findings do not contradict an *H. pylori*-positive diagnosis.

Corpus erosion

Description

Erosion in the corpus is found in both *H. pylori*-positive and negative cases. While it is somewhat more prevalent in *H. pylori*-negative cases, there is no significant difference[1]. According to a multicenter study, the accuracy rate for an *H. pylori*-negative diagnosis was 70% when flat erosion was recognized in the corpus, while the accuracy rate was 50% with raised erosion.

With regard to post-eradication conditions, no major studies have been conducted into corpus erosion. However, when the entire region is considered — not just the corpus — reports indicate that there were significantly more flat erosions after successful *H. pylori* eradication[2]. In other words, successful eradication results in the emergence of new erosions. It is believed that this is due to the restoration of gastric acid secretion possibly caused by successful eradication[2]. The emergence of new erosions after eradication together with the disappearance of infection findings in the background mucosa may endoscopically suggest successful eradication.

There appear to be three main types of corpus erosion: ① longitudinal or linear erosion located on the crest (ridge) of a fold or extending lengthwise along the extension line (**Fig. 1**); ② raised erosion on a fold or on the extension line (**Figs. 2 & 3**); and ③ erosion that emerges longitudinally (or in a longitudinal arrangement) on the lesser curvature side (**Figs. 4 & 5**).

The first type (①) is sometimes called crest erosion. When multiple raised erosions are lined up on a fold in the second type (②), they look like the suckers on octopus tentacles, so in Japan this type of erosion is referred to as octopus-sucker erosion. As it is also generated on the crests of folds and on their extension lines, it can also be called crest erosion. Among the third type of erosion (③), the type that forms a continuously linear shape in the longitudinal direction is sometimes called corpus linear erosion (**Fig. 4**). Unlike the first type (①), corpus linear erosion (③) is often generated on the opposite side (lesser curvature side) of the folds on the greater curvature side and accompanied by longitudinal redness (ridge-like redness) that looks as if it were mirroring the folds. Erosion appears in parts of the red area.

References

1) Kato T, Yagi N, Kamada T, et al ; Study Group for Establishing Endoscopic Diagnosis of Chronic Gastritis : Diagnosis of *Helicobacter pylori* infection in gastric mucosa by endoscopic features : a multicenter prospective study. Dig Endosc 2013 ; 25 : 508-518
2) Kato M, Terao S, Adachi K, et al ; Study Group for Establishing Endoscopic Diagnosis of Chronic Gastritis : Changes in endoscopic findings of gastritis after cure of *H. pylori* infection : multicenter prospective trial. Dig Endosc 2013 ; 25 : 264-273

17 Patchy redness

Masashi Kawamura

📖 Description ▶▶ Page 87

Fig. 1 Patchy redness accompanied by atrophic gastritis seen in an *H. pylori*-positive case

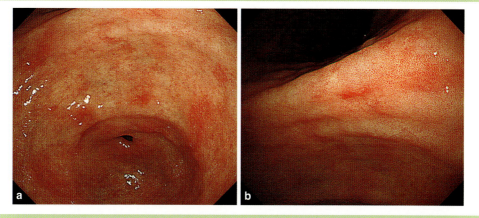

Fig. 2 Patchy redness in an *H. pylori*-positive case

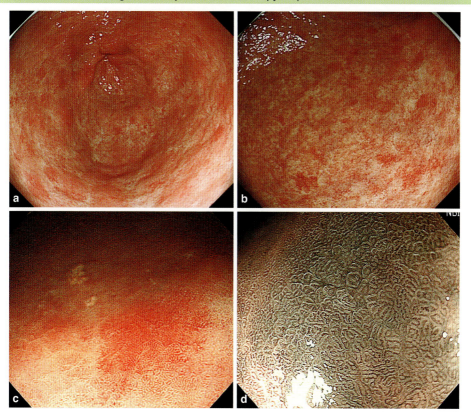

a, b: Patchy redness in the corpus and antrum seen in an *H. pylori*-positive case. **c:** In close-up/magnifying observation, flat redness with a faint margin can be seen. **d:** In magnifying Narrow Band Imaging (NBI) endoscopy, a flat image with an unclear margin accompanied by a minor change in the surface structure can be seen. [Structure Enhancement: B8; Color Enhancement: 1]

Chapter 2 Endoscopic Findings of Gastritis

Fig. 3 Patchy redness after *H. pylori* eradication (1)

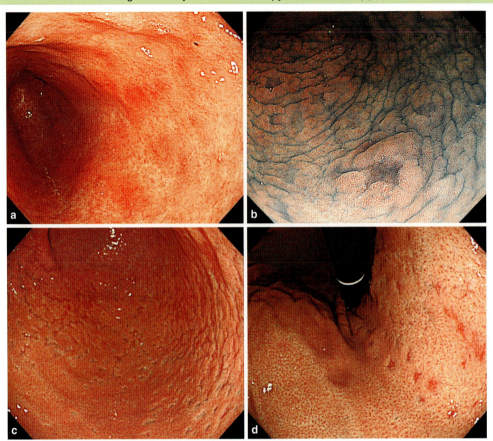

a: Patchy redness in the antrum seen after *H. pylori* eradication.
b: After spraying with indigo carmine, multiple depressions with clear margins can be seen.
c, d: Patchy redness with clear margins and depressions can be seen in the corpus.

- Equipment used (Pages 83–86)
  Endoscopes: GIF-H260 (Figs. 1, 5 & 7); GIF-H260Z (Figs. 2–4); GIF-Q260 (Fig. 6) (Olympus)
  Light source: EVIS LUCERA SPECTRUM CLV-260SL (Olympus)

2. Specific Discussions ● 85

Fig. 4   Patchy redness after *H. pylori* eradication (2)

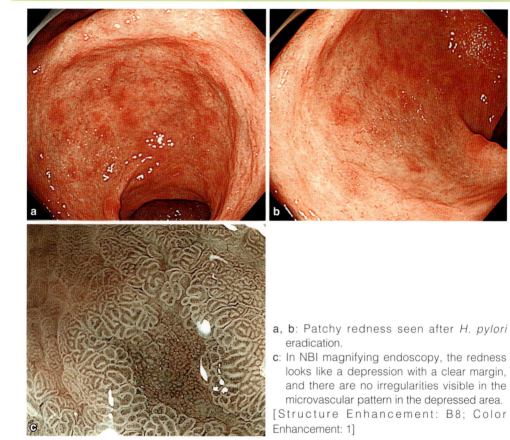

a, b: Patchy redness seen after *H. pylori* eradication.
c: In NBI magnifying endoscopy, the redness looks like a depression with a clear margin, and there are no irregularities visible in the microvascular pattern in the depressed area.
[Structure Enhancement: B8; Color Enhancement: 1]

Fig. 5   Patchy redness in the antrum seen in a patient taking low-dose aspirin medication

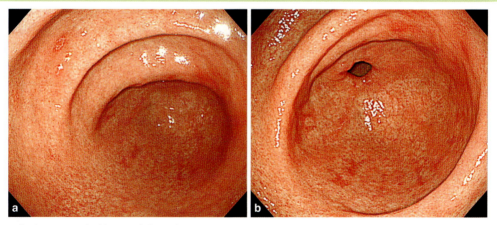

a, b: Accompanied by partial erosion.

Fig. 6 Patchy redness in the antrum and corpus seen in a patient taking NSAIDs

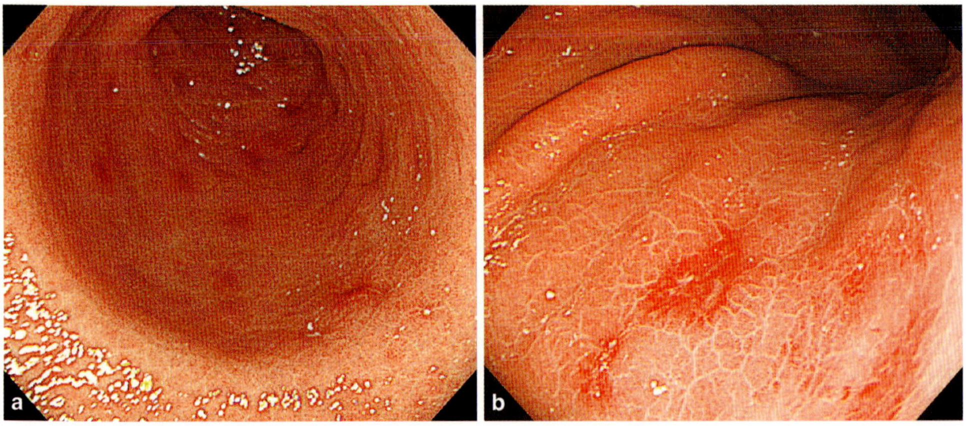

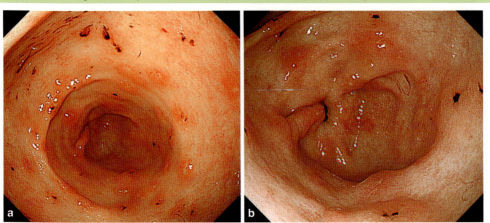

a: In the antrum, redness is seen here and there.
b: Patchy redness in the corpus is accompanied by erosion.

Fig. 7 Patchy redness in the antrum seen in a patient taking NSAIDs

a, b: Accompanied by partial erosion and attachment of hematin.

Patchy redness

Description

Patchy redness is an oval erythema finding on the gastric mucosa that can be seen in endoscopy[1), 2)].

In addition to endoscopic atrophy of the gastric mucosa, patchy redness accompanied by chronic gastritis caused by *H. pylori* infection is apparent in multiple locations in the region from the antrum to the corpus. It looks like flat redness with an indistinct margin (**Figs. 1 & 2**).

Patchy redness is also seen on the gastric mucosa after *H. pylori* eradication. The patchy redness seen after eradication often exhibits a clearer margin and slightly more depressed shape than the patchy redness that appears during *H. pylori* infection. In some cases, an extensive map-like redness also appears in the corpus (**Figs. 3 & 4**) (see 18 "Map-like redness"). Patchy redness (mottled patchy erythema) has also been reported after eradication and has been correlated with intestinal metaplasia[3)]. It is believed to be an important finding for *H. pylori*-post infected cases.

Gastric mucosal damage caused by drugs such as low-dose aspirin and NSAIDs[4), 5)] can also produce patchy redness regardless of *H. pylori* infection. The patchy redness caused by medications such as low-dose aspirin and NSAIDs is occasionally accompanied by hematin, erosions, and ulcers (**Figs. 5–7**). In some cases of drug-induced patchy redness, the condition clears up when the patient stops taking the medication.

As has been pointed out, patchy redness is seen in all types of cases — those not infected with *H. pylori*, as well as those with a current infection or past infection. Consequently, the presence or absence of patchy redness is not helpful in diagnosing the state of *H. pylori* infection. Nonetheless, because patchy redness exhibits variable endoscopic characteristics depending on its cause, it is important to have an understanding of the morphologies it takes and the margins it forms when observing the characteristics of patchy redness.

Another type of redness that needs to be differentiated endoscopically from patchy redness is spotty redness. This is commonly seen during *H. pylori* infection and appears as smaller dots than patchy redness, tending to aggregate in the region from the corpus to the fornix. Enlarged capillaries and small hyperplastic polyps may also look similar to patchy redness when viewed endoscopically, so it is important to differentiate them.

References

1) Kaminishi M, Yamaguchi H, Nomura S, et al : Endoscopic classification of chronic gastritis based on a pilot study by the research society for gastritis. Dig Endosc 2002 ; 14 : 138-151
2) Nomura S, Terao S, Adachi K, et al : Endoscopic diagnosis of gastric mucosal activity and inflammation. Dig Endosc 2013 ; 25 : 136-146
3) Nagata N, Shimbo T, Akiyama J, et al : Predictability of gastric intestinal metaplasia by mottled patchy erythema seen on endoscopy. Gastroenterology Research 2011 ; 4 : 203-209
4) Iwamoto J, Mizokami Y, Shimokobe K, et al : Clinical features of gastroduodenal ulcer in Japanese patients taking low-dose aspirin. Dig Dis Sci 2010 ; 55 : 2270-2274
5) Huang JQ, Sridhar S and Hunt RH : Role of infection and non-steroidal anti-inflammatory drugs in peptic-ulcer disease : a meta-analysis. Lancet 2002 ; 359 (9300) : 14-22

88 • Chapter 2 Endoscopic Findings of Gastritis

18 Map-like redness

Mitsugi Yasuda

📖 Description ▶▶ Page 90

Fig. 1 Map-like redness in the antrum

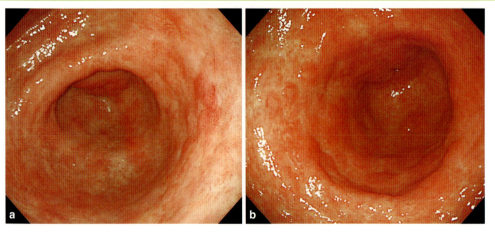

a: Map-like redness that emerges on the atrophic gastric mucosa in the antrum.
b: Patchy redness adheres and forms a map-like pattern.

Fig. 2 Map-like redness (1)

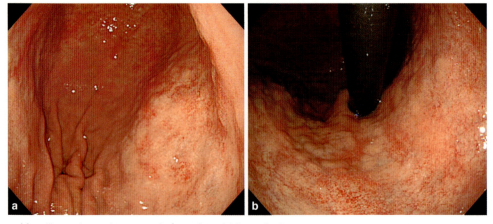

a: Map-like redness that extends from the middle to the lower corpus.
b: Map-like redness from the upper corpus to the cardia.

• Equipment used (Pages 88–89)
  Endoscope: GIF-H260 (Olympus)
  Light source: EVIS LUCERA (Olympus)

Fig. 3 Map-like redness (2)

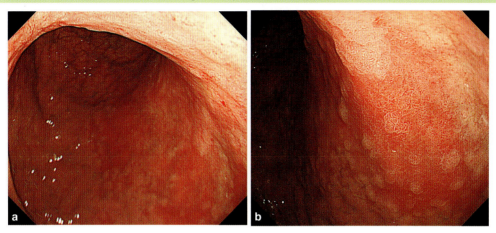

a: Typical map-like redness with relatively clear margins.
b: Close-up image of typical map-like redness. It is slightly depressed compared to its surroundings.

Fig. 4 Before and after *H. pylori* eradication

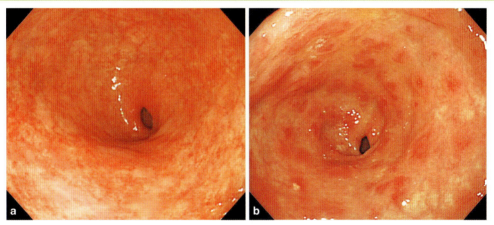

Before eradication   After eradication

a: Finding of atrophy and intestinal metaplasia in the antrum (before eradication).
b: Map-like redness has emerged in the antrum (after eradication).

Map-like redness

📖 Description

Map-like redness is a characteristic finding that emerges after the eradication of *H. pylori*[1,2].

The basic endoscopic finding in *H. pylori* infection is diffuse redness. In some cases, however, patchy redness emerges after diffuse redness has disappeared due to eradication. These patches can vary in size and shape, but they have clearer margins than the patchy redness seen during *H. pylori* infection and tend to be slightly depressed. The patches are larger than the spotty redness seen in the upper corpus. Patches of redness 5 to 10-mm in size appear in the center of the antrum (**Fig. 1**), together with larger areas of map-like redness. The intensity of the redness can also vary ranging from weak (**Fig. 2**) to strong (**Fig. 3**).

In histological examination using biopsy specimens, findings of intestinal metaplasia are often obtained. This is believed to be caused by the enhancement of the intestinal metaplastic areas due to changes in the intragastric environment subsequent to eradication. **Fig. 4** shows a case where atrophy and intestinal metaplasia can be seen in the antrum and map-like redness has emerged following eradication.

Map-like redness is not always found following eradication. However, when it is observed, there is virtually no doubt that it is indicative of post-eradication gastric mucosa.

References

1) Nagata N, Shimbo T, Akiyama J, et al : Predictability of gastric intestinal metaplasia by mottled patchy erythema seen on endoscopy. Gastroenterology Research 2011 ; 4 : 203-209
2) Watanabe K, Nagata N, Nakashima R, et al : Predictive findings for *Helicobacter pylori*-uninfected, -infected and -eradicated gastric mucosa : Validation study. World J Gastroenterol 2013 ; 19 : 4374-4379

2. Specific Discussions • 91

19 Multiple white and flat elevated lesions

Tomoari Kamada

📖 Description ▶▶ Page 93

Fig. 1 Multiple white and flat elevated lesions (1)

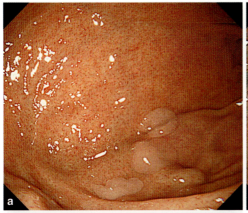
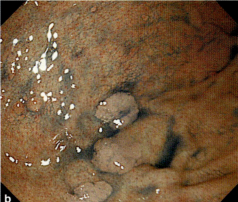
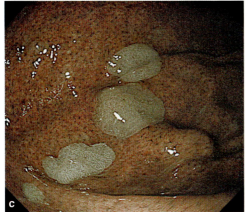

70s, female. Following long-term administration of a PPI due to reflux esophagitis, white and flat elevated lesions have appeared in multiple locations on the greater curvature of the fornix.
a: Conventional observation image.
b: Indigo carmine sprayed observation.
c: NBI observation.
d: Biopsy tissue collected from a white and flat elevated lesion (low magnification, HE-stained).
e: Same tissue (high magnification, HE- stained). Hyperplastic change can be seen in the fundic gland foveolar epithelium.

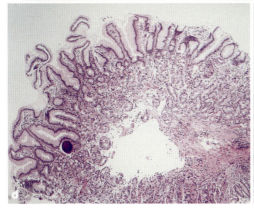
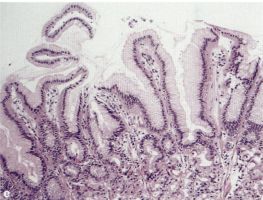

Fig. 2 Multiple white and flat elevated lesions (2)

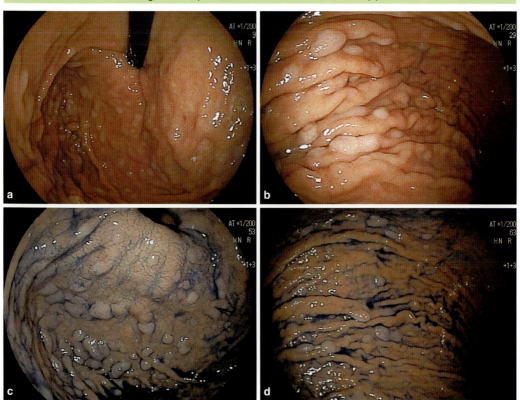

80s, female, following long-term administration of a PPI due to reflux esophagitis.
a, b: Multiple white and flat elevated lesions in the region from the corpus to the greater curvature of the fornix can be seen in conventional observation.
c, d: Indigo-carmine spraying has made the lesions clearer.

Fig. 3 Multiple white and flat elevated lesions (3)

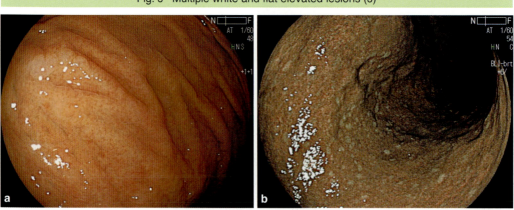

White and flat elevated lesions have emerged in multiple locations in the greater curvature of the corpus (under PPI administration)
a: Conventional observation image.
b: The white and flat elevated lesions are noticeably clearer in BLI-bright mode.

- Equipment used (Pages 91–93)
  Endoscopes: GIF-H260 (Olympus); EG-L590ZW (Fujifilm); etc.
  Light sources: EVIS LUCERA, etc. (Olympus); LASEREO, etc. (Fujifilm)

Fig. 3 Continued

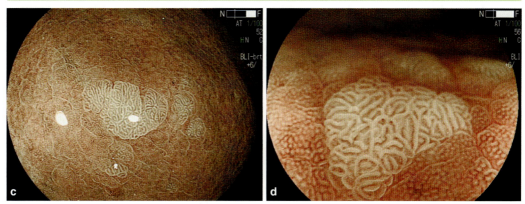

c: Medium-magnification image in BLI-bright mode.
d: High-magnification image in BLI-bright mode. The surface structure exhibits a tubular pattern.

Multiple white and flat elevated lesions

Description

Until recently only a few studies noted the appearance of whitish flat lesions in multiple locations from the upper corpus to the fornix. In a study entitled "Investigation into Multiple White and Flat Elevated Lesions Found in the Gastric Body"[1] presented at the 73rd Congress of the Japan Gastroenterological Endoscopy Society, Kawaguchi et al. reported 20 clinical cases. In these cases, the occurrence rate was higher in females than in males — with a male-to-female ratio of approximately 7:13. The mean age was 68.1 (38 to 92). In 13 out of 20 cases (65%), a proton pump inhibitor (PPI) or H_2 receptor antagonist had been administered.

Since this report, it has become clear that white and flat elevated lesions occur in multiple locations at a high rate when the region from the upper corpus to the fornix is carefully observed, especially in patients who have been taking PPIs[2]. When the region from the upper corpus to the greater curvature of the fornix is observed, whitish and flat elevations of various sizes can be seen in multiple locations (**Figs. 1 & 2**). When observed from distance, these lesions may not always be visible. However, it is possible to accurately diagnose them by bringing the distal end of the endoscope up close or using image enhanced endoscopy (IEE) such as Narrow Band Imaging (NBI), Flexible spectral Imaging Color Enhancement (FICE), and Blue Laser Imaging (BLI) (**Fig. 3**). The characteristics of the endoscopic findings are flat elevations of various sizes with a whitish color tone and low height. The surface of the elevation does not have a dilated vascular pattern like that seen in fundic gland polyps. When observed up close, tubular patterns can be seen. Histologically, hyperplastic changes in the foveolar epithelium are recognized (**Fig. 1c**). Currently, long-term administration of PPIs is applicable mainly to reflux esophagitis patients. The occurrence frequency of multiple white and flat elevated lesions (Haruma-Kawaguchi lesions) is expected to increase in the future.

References

1) Kawaguchi M, Arai E, Nozawa H, et al. : [Investigation into multiple white and flat elevated lesions found in the corpus.] Gastroenterol Endosc 2007; 49 (Suppl 1): 958 (In Japanese)
2) Haruma K, Shiotani A, Kamata T, et al. : [Adverse effects induced by long-term use of proton pump inhibitors — development of gastric polyps.] Shokakinaika 2013; 56: 190-193 (In Japanese)

Additional Information

Cobblestone Mucosa

Tomoari Kamada

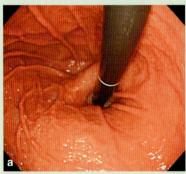
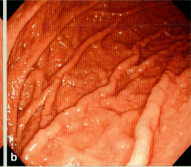

Fig. 1 Patient with long-term administration of PPI due to reflux esophagitis
Cobblestone mucosa in the corpus mucosa.
a: Retrograde view of the corpus.
b: Forward view of the corpus.

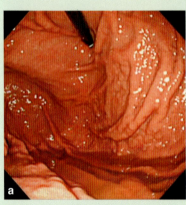
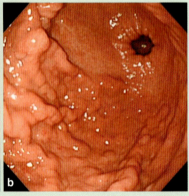

Fig. 2 Observation using an ultraslim endoscope
Cobblestone mucosa in the corpus.
a: Retrograde view of the corpus.
b: Forward view of the corpus.

Occasionally, the mucosa in the gastric body looks as cobblestones, this finding is called cobblestone mucosa. Cobblestone mucosa is almost the same color as the background mucosa and is mainly composed of numerous small granular elevations. Many of these elevations are seen between folds, giving the gastric mucosa a lumpy appearance.

This type of gastritis has rarely been reported and is distinguished by the fact that there is no *H. pylori* infection and that in many cases a proton pump inhibitor (PPI) has been administered for long-term periods (**Figs. 1 & 3**). Because the PPI combines with the proton pump in the gastric parietal cells to suppress gastric acid secretion, long-term use of a PPI causes hyperplastic changes and deformations in the gastric parietal cells known as hypergastrinemia, resulting in the emergence of the elevations.

Another type of mucosal change in the corpus induced by PPIs is the appearance of white and flat elevated lesions. Because they are multiple low and flat elevations, whitish in color, and in a wide range of sizes, this type of mucosal change can easily be differentiated from cobblestone mucosa.

Reference
1) Haruma K, Shiotani A, Kamada T, et al. : [Adverse effects induced by long-term use of proton pump inhibitors — development of gastric polyps.] Shokakinaika 2013; 56: 190–193 (In Japanese)

2. Specific Discussions ● 95

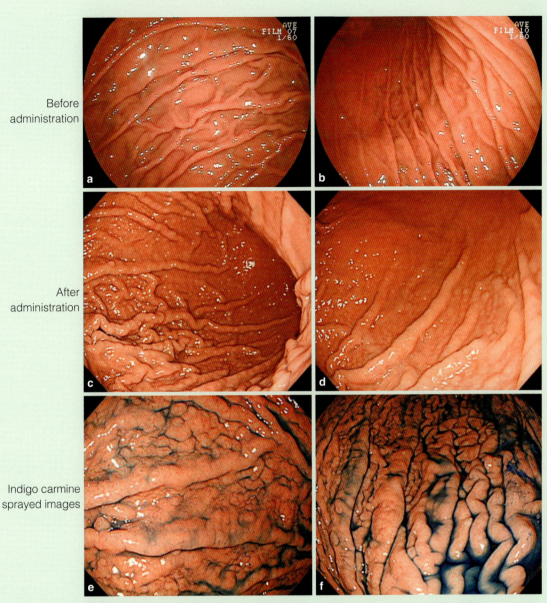

Fig. 3　A case of cobblestone mucosa (before and after administration of a PPI)
  a, b: Before PPI administration. The corpus mucosa is smooth and there is no sign of cobblestone mucosa.
  c, d: After PPI administration. Cobblestone mucosa can be seen in the corpus.
  e, f: Indigo carmine sprayed images. The cobblestone mucosa between the folds is clearer.

Chapter 3

Endoscopic Findings for Risk Stratification of Gastric Cancer

Chapter 3   Endoscopic Findings for Risk Stratification of Gastric Cancer

1. Description

Mototsugu Kato

The Kyoto Classification of Gastritis is divided into categories to facilitate diagnosis of findings of endoscopic gastritis and to evaluate the risk of gastric cancer. The former categories are discussed in detail in Chapter 2. In this chapter, we will discuss how those findings can be used for risk stratification of gastric cancer.

1 Relationship between gastric cancer and background gastritis

Gastric cancer is among a number of cancers that tend to develop against a background of chronic disease — in this case, gastritis. The relationship between *H. pylori* and gastric cancer is similar to the relationships between viral hepatitis and liver cancer, ulcerative colitis and colitic cancer, or reflex esophagitis and esophageal adenocarcinoma; that is, carcinogenesis is induced by the accumulation of genetic abnormalities as a result of chronic inflammation. Both differentiated and undifferentiated gastric cancers are generated from inflammatory mucosa infected with *H. pylori*. Where gastric mucosa has never been infected by *H. pylori*, the rate of gastric cancer is thought to occupy less than 1%. A prospective study conducted in Europe reported that 15-year follow-up observations found gastric cancer in roughly 10% of atrophic gastritis patients, while no cancer was found in the non-atrophic control group[1]. A similar prospective study based on periodic endoscopic examinations was conducted in Japan[2].

While *H. pylori* infection is the most common cause of gastritis, there is another type of gastritis known as autoimmune type A gastritis which is relatively rare in Japan. When the gastric mucosa is infected with *H. pylori*, inflammatory cells begin to accumulate in the lamina propria of the gastric mucosa. These cells are immunocompetent lymphocytes and plasma cells that secrete immunoglobulins. They are also accompanied by polynuclear neutrophils. As a result of lymphocyte accumulation, lymph follicle formation, gastric mucosal epithelium damage, proliferative and hyperplastic changes in the mucosal epithelium, etc., the processes of destruction and regeneration are repeated again and again. Eventually, the proper gastric glands disappear and pseudopyloric gland metaplasia and intestinal metaplasia emerge, becoming atrophic gastritis. Chronic gastritis is divided into three types according to the location of the inflammation: antrum-predominant gastritis, pangastritis, and corpus-predominant gastritis (**Fig. 1**)[3]. The onset of related diseases is closely associated with to the type of gastritis. In antrum-predominant gastritis, acid secretion increases, eventually leading to a duodenal ulcer and only rarely in gastric carcinogenesis. In pangastritis, inflammation expands to the corpus and can become a

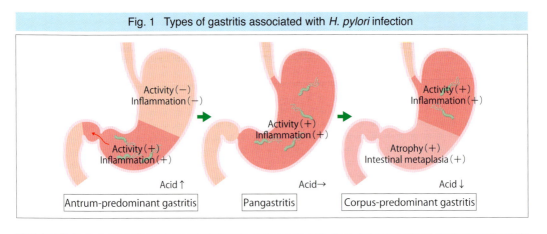

Fig. 1 Types of gastritis associated with *H. pylori* infection

Fig. 2 OLGA staging and OLGIM staging

Risk level of gastric cancer	Corpus (pathology)			
	No atrophy	Mild atrophy	Moderate atrophy	Severe atrophy
Antrum(pathology) — No atrophy	Stage 0	Stage I	Stage II	Stage III
Antrum(pathology) — Mild atrophy	Stage I	Stage I	Stage II	Stage III
Antrum(pathology) — Moderate atrophy	Stage II	Stage II	Stage III	Stage IV
Antrum(pathology) — Severe atrophy	Stage III	Stage III	Stage IV	Stage IV

Risk level of gastric cancer	Corpus (pathology)			
	No IM	Mild IM	Moderate IM	Severe IM
Antrum(pathology) — No IM	Stage 0	Stage I	Stage II	Stage III
Antrum(pathology) — Mild IM	Stage I	Stage I	Stage II	Stage III
Antrum(pathology) — Moderate IM	Stage II	Stage II	Stage III	Stage IV
Antrum(pathology) — Severe IM	Stage III	Stage III	Stage IV	Stage IV

IM：intestinal metaplasia
Lowest (stage 0) to highest (stage IV)

OLGA staging
[Rugge M, et al：Gut　2007；56：631-636[4]]

OLGIM staging
[Capelle LG, et al：Gastrointest Endosc 2010;71：1150-1158[5]]

premalignant lesion of undifferentiated cancer. Corpus-predominant gastritis causes atrophic changes to expand to the gastric body, reducing acid secretion, and can develop into gastric ulcers or differentiated adenocarcinoma[2]. Because corpus-predominant gastritis is common among East Asian people including Korean and a subset of Chinese, *H. pylori*-infected patients in Japan and Korea frequently end up with atrophic gastritis, suggesting that atrophy and intestinal metaplasia — especially with incomplete-type intestinal metaplasia — are closely related to the occurrence of differentiated gastric cancer. Nevertheless, no evidence has been found that clearly shows that adenocarcinoma is generated from intestinal metaplastic glandular ducts. Clinical investigations thus far have however showed clearly that there is a high risk of differentiated adenocarcinoma developing from background mucosa with intestinal metaplasia.

Two gastritis staging systems — OLGA (Operative Link on Gastritis Assessment) and OLGIM (Operative Link on Gastric Intestinal Metaplasia assessment) — can be used to assess the risk of gastric cancer depending on the degree of pathological atrophy and intestinal metaplasia in the gastric antrum and corpus (**Fig. 2**). In a case-control study using these staging systems, a significant correlation was found between OLGIM staging and gastric cancer. The study found that the cancer risk for corpus predominant gastritis was 3.4 (1.4–8.1). However, when evaluated in combination with OLGIM staging, the odds ratio increased to 9.8 (2.6–36.7) — based on the scores of endoscopic findings used to assess the risk of gastric cancer[6].

2 Endoscopic findings related to the risk of gastric cancer

In a case control study conducted in Japan, endoscopic findings related to the risk of gastric cancer — such as the degree and extent of atrophy, redness, and granular changes — were investigated. The risk of gastric cancer with atrophic gastritis was 5.13 (2.79–9.42). The odds ratio of differentiated cancer jumped to 24.71 (3.46–176.68) with severe atrophy while remaining low at 3.49 (1.77–6.89) for undifferentiated cancer. Endoscopic findings such as redness or granular changes did not appear to increase the risk of gastric cancer. Atrophic changes, on the other hand, played a major role in the generation of gastric cancer[7]. Another study looked at the correlation between endoscopic screening for gastric cancer in medical checkups and the frequency rate for discovery of gastric cancer over the following 11 years. The study clearly showed that increases in the frequency of gastric cancer were closely correlated with the progress of gastric mucosal atrophy[8]. With endoscopic atrophic scores of C-0 and C-1 the gastric cancer frequency rate was 0%, while with C-2 and C-3 the rate was 2.2%, with O-1 and O-2 it was 4.4%, and with O-3 and O-p it was 10.3%[8].

Nodular gastritis is special type of gastritis distinguished by lymphoid follicle formation associated with *H. pylori* infection. Endoscopically, it is characterized by multiple small elevations with white crests that appear mainly in the pyloric antrum. It is known that nodular gastritis poses a risk of gastric cancer in young females — predominantly undifferentiated cancer — with an odds ratio of 64.2[9]. A study using gastric X-ray images reported that enlarged (hypertrophic) folds in the gastric body could be a risk factor for undifferentiated cancer — although endoscopy was not used. According to this study, when the risk of cancer was set to 1 for folds with a width of less than 4 mm, the risk of gastric cancer increased to 3.1 for folds with a width of 5 mm, to 8.6 with a width of 6 mm, and to 35.5 with a width of 7 mm[10].

3 Scores for endoscopic findings related to the risk of gastric cancer

Based on this analysis, we designated atrophy, intestinal metaplasia, fold enlargement (hypertrophy), and nodularity as endoscopic findings that can be used in assessing the risk of gastric cancer. We also selected diffuse redness as a finding that can be used to distinguish between conditions during *H. pylori* infection and after *H. pylori* eradication — something that is important when considering the gastric cancer suppression effect of *H. pylori* eradication. More precisely, if eradication has eliminated inflammatory cell infiltration and the gastric mucosa has recovered to a state equivalent to uninfected mucosa (**Table 1**), the risk of gastric cancer is further decreased.

102 ● Chapter 3 Endoscopic Findings for Risk Stratification of Gastric Cancer

Table 1 Grading endoscopic findings related to gastric cancer risk

● **Atrophy**: Do not distinguish between WLI and IEE.
　　A → 0 (None C-0 or C-1), 1 (Minor C-2 or C-3), 2 (Severe O-1 to O-P)
● **Intestinal metaplasia**: Distinguish between WLI and IEE.
　　　※ In IEE (NBI, BLI, etc.) evaluate the degree and extent of LBC and WOS.
　　　※ In IEE, enter the score in parentheses but do not include it in the total — e.g., $IM_{1(2)}$
　　IM → 0 (Absence), 1 (Antrum), 2 (Antrum/Corpus)
● **Fold enlargement** (hypertrophy)
　　H → 0 (Absence), 1 (Presence)
● **Nodularity**
　　N → 0 (Absence), 1 (Presence)
● **Diffuse redness** (visibility of vascular patterns of collecting venules in the corpus gland region):
　　　　　　Changes after the eradication should also be taken into consideration.
　　DR → 0 (None), 1 (Minor: Partially RAC+), 2 (Severe)

★ Entry method: Indicate all factors and enter the total score in the final
parentheses (min. 0 to max. 8).
　　E.g., A_1 IM_1 H_1 N_1 $DR_{2(6)}$

● Atrophy (A)

No distinction should be made between WLI endoscopy and image enhancement endoscopy (IEE). Enter a score of 0 for C-0 and C-1 where no atrophy is recognized, score 1 point for C-2 and C-3 where atrophy is minor, and score 2 points for O-1 to O-P where atrophy is moderate to severe. For example, enter A1 when the score is 1.

● Intestinal metaplasia (IM)

Intestinal metaplasia looks completely different when viewed in standard WLI observation than under IEE observation. In WLI, observation shows only white elevated lesions, which are referred to as special type of intestinal metaplasia. After *H. pylori* eradication, reddish depressed lesions can be seen. On the other hand, under chromoendoscopy using methylene blue, various intestinal metaplastic lesions can be observed, in addition to the special type. When intestinal metaplasia is observed with short-wavelength narrow-band light such as NBI and BLI, light blue crests (LBCs) with margins of pale blue-white light can be observed on the surface of the foveolar epithelium. Moreover, under NBI and BLI, special type of intestinal metaplasia shows up as a white opaque substance (WOS) that looks as if it is attached to the mucosal epithelium. The degree and extent of LBCs and WOS should be evaluated under IEE observation. Hence, WLI and IEE observation data should be entered separately.

If intestinal metaplasia is not recognized, enter a score of 0. When intestinal metaplasia can be seen in the antrum, enter a score of 1. When intestinal metaplasia extends to the gastric body, enter a score of 2. Score 1 should be written down as "IM_1" for WLI observation data and in parentheses for IEE observation data. For example, when the score is 1 in WLI observation and 2 in IEE observation, enter "$IM_{1(2)}$".

● Fold enlargement (hypertrophy)

When the width of a fold is 4 mm or less in observation with sufficient insufflation, enter a score of 0. When it is 5 mm or more, enter a score of 1 and write down "H_1".

● Nodularity

When there is no nodularity, enter a score of 0. If nodularity is observed, enter a score of 1

Table 2 Grading endoscopic findings for gastric cancer risk and estimated scores according to disease (example)

Non-infected patient	$=0$
Antrum-predominant gastritis	$=1$
Pangastritis without atrophy (including nodularity)cc	$=2$ to 4
Atrophic gastritis (corpus-predominant gastritis)	$=3$ to 8
Post-eradication case	$=-1$ to -2

and write down "N_1".

● **Diffuse redness**

Observe the areas of the corpus glands where there is no atrophy. If the endoscopist is not familiar with this observation, it is a good idea to diagnose diffuseness using vascular patterns of collecting venules in the corpus grand region. When RAC is recognized, it means that there is no diffuse redness, so enter a score of 0. When RAC has disappeared, enter a score of 2. When some RAC is visible after *H. pylori* eradication, enter a score of 1. Write down "DR_2" when the score is 2, for example.

All risk factors are entered — for example, as A_1 $IM_{1\,(2)}$ H_0 N_1 DR_2. The total score is put in parentheses at the end of the risk factors— for example, as A_1 $IM_{1\,(2)}$ H_0 N_1 $DR_{2\,(5)}$. The total score ranges from a minimum of 0 to a maximum of 8 (**Table 2**).

Conclusion

The gastric cancer risk classification discussed in this chapter was created by selecting known endoscopic findings related to cancer risk and scoring them accordingly. It is important to make clear that the evidence supporting this classification is not yet sufficient and that it is necessary to verify this gastritis risk classification by applying it in actual clinical cases. Depending on the results of the verification, it may be necessary to change the scoring system. We look forward to seeing this classification used as a basis for further study.

References

1) Cheli R, Santi L, Ciancamerla G, et al：A clinical and statistical follow-up study of atrophic gastritis. Am J Dig Dis　1973；18：1061-1065
2) Uemura N, Okamoto S, Yamamoto S, et al：*Helicobacter pylori* infection and the development of gastric cancer. N Engl J Med　2001；345：784-789
3) Price AB：The Sydney System：Histological division. J Gastroenterol Hepatol　1991；6：209-222
4) Rugge M, Meggio A, Pennelli G, et al：Gastritis staging in clinical practice：the OLGA staging system. Gut　2007；56：631-636
5) Capelle LG, de Vries AC, Haringsma J, et al：The staging of gastritis with the OLGA system by using intestinal metaplasia as an accurate alternative for atrophic gastritis. Gastrointest Endosc 2010；71：1150-1158
6) Tsai YC, Hsiao WH, Yang HB, et al：The corpus-predominant gastritis index may serve as an early marker of *Helicobacter pylori*-infected patients at risk of gastric cancer. Aliment Pharmacol Ther　2013；37：969-978
7) Kato I, Tominaga S, Ito Y, et al：Atrophic gastritis and stomach cancer risk：cross-sectional analyses. Jpn J Cancer Res　1992；83：1041-1046
8) Inoue K, Fujisawa T, Chinuki D, et al：[Background mucosa for gastric cancer occurrence: investigation with endoscopy in medical checkups.] I to Cho (Stomach Intest)　2009; 44: 1367–1373 (In Japanese)
9) Kamada T, Tanaka A, Yamanaka Y, et al：Nodular gastritis with *Helicobacter pylori* infection is strongly associated with diffuse-type gastric cancer in young patients. Dig Endosc　2007；19：180-184
10) Nishibayashi H, Kanayama S, Kiyohara T, et al：*Helicobacter pylori*-induced enlarged-fold gastritis is associated with increased mutagenicity of gastric juice, increased oxidative DNA damage, and an increased risk of gastric carcinoma. J Gastroenterol Hepatol　2003；18：1384-1391

Chapter 3 Endoscopic Findings for Risk Stratification of Gastric Cancer

2. Clinical Cases

Tomoari Kamada

Case 1 (before eradication treatment)

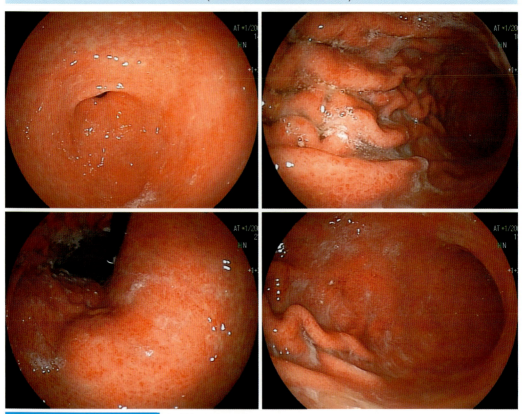

Endoscopic finding scores A₁ IM₀ H₁ N₀ DR₂ (4)

[Description]
Atrophy (Kimura–Takemoto Classification Type C-3): A₁
Intestinal metaplasia absent: IM₀
Fold enlargement (hypertrophy) Present: H₁
Nodularity absent: N₀
Severe diffuse redness: DR₂
Total score: 4

Case 1 (1 year after eradication)

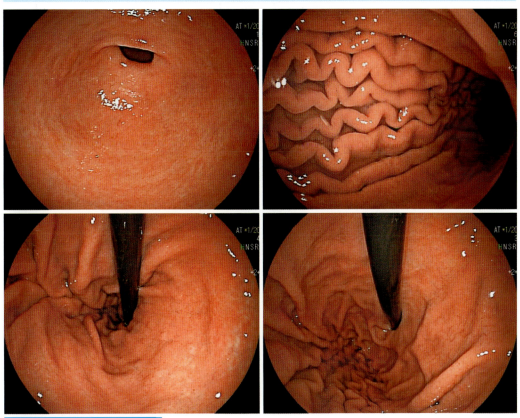

Endoscopic finding scores   A₁ IM₀ H₀ N₀ DR₀ (1)

[Description]
Atrophy (Kimura-Takemoto Classification Type C-3): A₁
Intestinal metaplasia absent: IM₀
Fold enlargement (hypertrophy) absent: H₀
Nodularity absent: N₀
Diffuse redness absent: DR₀
Total score: 1
The endoscopic finding scores improved 1 year after eradication.

106 • Chapter 3 Endoscopic Findings for Risk Stratification of Gastric Cancer

Case 2

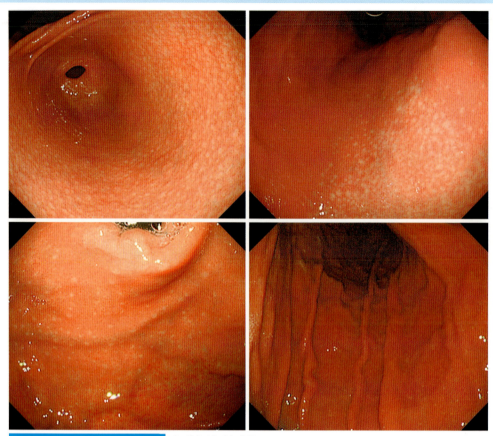

Endoscopic finding scores A₁ IM₀ H₀ N₁ DR₂ (4)

[Description]
Atrophy (Kimura–Takemoto Classification Type C-3): A₁
Intestinal metaplasia absent: IM₀
Fold enlargement (hypertrophy) absent: H₀
Nodularity Present: N₁
Severe diffuse redness: DR₂
Total score: 4

Case 3

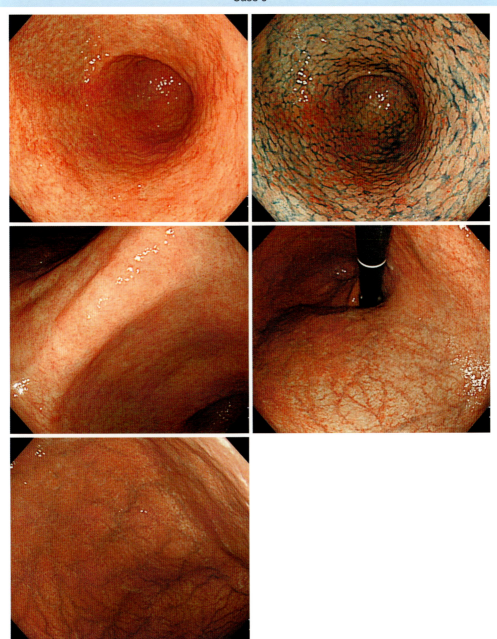

Endoscopic finding scores A₂ IM₁ H₀ N₀ DR₂ (5)

[Description]
Atrophy (Kimura-Takemoto Classification Type O-2): A₂
Intestinal metaplasia Present only in antrum: IM₁
Fold enlargement (hypertrophy) absent: H₀
Nodularity absent: N₀
Severe diffuse redness: DR₂
Total score: 5

Case 4

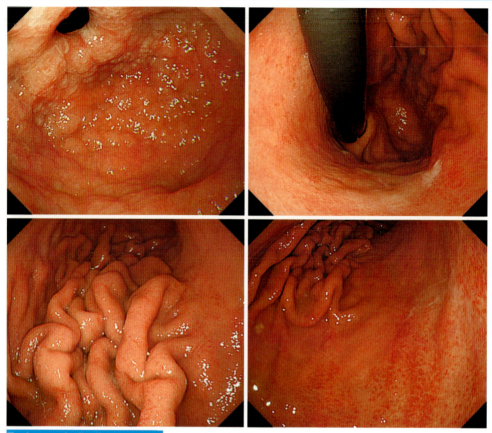

Endoscopic finding scores   A₂ IM₁ H₁ N₀ DR₂ (6)

[Description]
Atrophy (Kimura-Takemoto Classification Type O-1): A₂
Intestinal metaplasia Present only in antrum: IM₁
Fold enlargement (hypertrophy) Present: H₁
Nodularity absent: N₀
Severe diffuse redness: DR₂
Total score: 6

Case 5

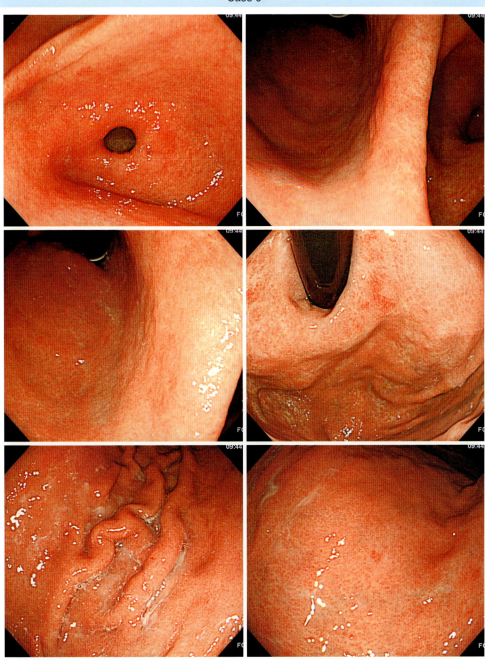

Endoscopic finding scores A$_2$ IM$_0$ H$_1$ N$_0$ DR$_2$ (5)

[Description]
Atrophy (Kimura-Takemoto Classification Type O-1): A$_2$
Intestinal metaplasia absent: IM$_0$
Fold enlargement (hypertrophy) Present: H$_1$
Nodularity absent: N$_0$
Severe diffuse redness: DR$_2$
Total score: 5

110 • Chapter 3 Endoscopic Findings for Risk Stratification of Gastric Cancer

Case 6

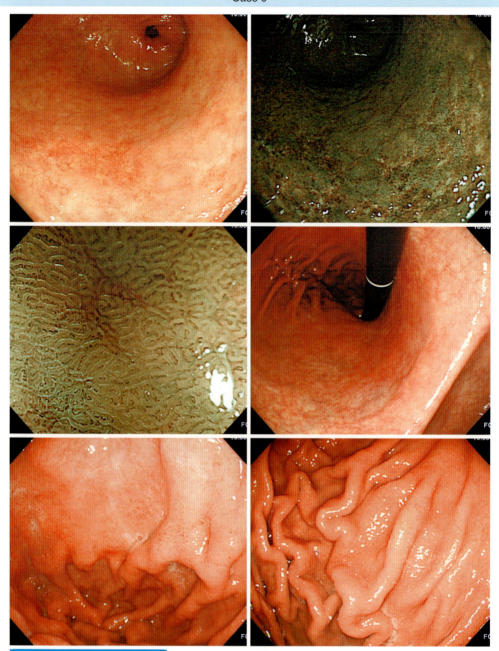

Endoscopic finding scores A₂ IM₁₍₁₎ H₁ N₀ DR₂ ₍₆₎

[Description]
Atrophy (Kimura-Takemoto Classification Type O-2): A₂
Intestinal metaplasia Presence (LBCs observed in NBI magnifying observation): IM₁₍₁₎
Fold enlargement (hypertrophy) Present: H₁
Nodularity absent: N₀
Severe diffuse redness: DR₂
Total score: 6

Chapter 4

Recording Endoscopic Findings of Gastritis

Chapter 4 Recording Endoscopic Findings of Gastritis

1. Description and Clinical Cases

Katsuhiro Mabe

 Basic method for entering data

Gastritis is associated with histological inflammation of the gastric mucosa and is usually caused by *Helicobacter pylori* (*H. pylori*) infection with the exception of autoimmune gastritis which is especially rare in Japan. The findings of histological gastritis are recorded using the Updated Sydney System (USS) (Fig. 3 on page 12), in which mononuclear infiltration, neutrophil infiltration, atrophy, intestinal metaplasia, and *H. pylori* infection in the corpus and antrum are rated in four stages: absent, mild, moderate, and severe[1]. Endoscopic findings, on the other hand, have still not been classified into a truly universal gastritis classification system. Schindler's Classification (for superficial, atrophic, and hypertrophic gastritis) proposed in 1947 remains the standard in the field. Although the USS sorts endoscopic findings into 11 items and endoscopic gastritis into 7 types, it is not widely used either because it is complicated, is not practical for clinical practice, and does not necessarily correspond with histological gastritis.

Thanks to the remarkable progress of endoscopic technology such as in HDTV, magnifying endoscopy, and image enhancement endoscopy (IEE), however, it is now required that *H. pylori* infection conditions — i.e., non-infection, current infection, and past infection — be endoscopically diagnosed, especially since eradication treatment of *H. pylori*-induced gastritis is now covered by the Japanese health insurance system.

In 2013, after conducting multicenter studies nationwide, the Study Group for the Establishment of Endoscopic Diagnosis of Chronic Gastritis, which is affiliated with the Japan Gastroenterological Endoscopy Society, announced the publication of two papers — one reporting on diagnosis of *H. pylori* infection by endoscopic features[2] and the other on changes in endoscopic findings before and after *H. pylori* eradication[3]. At the 85th Congress of the JGES, chaired by Dr. Haruma and held in Kyoto the same year, participants took part in spirited discussions at a symposium on the significance of endoscopic gastritis in the battle to defeat gastric cancer, as well as at a workshop dedicated to the preparation of the Updated Kyoto Classification — the new grading system for endoscopic gastritis.

New gastritis classification and gastric cancer risk evaluation systems are not issues that are discussed at a congress and then forgotten about. They are subjects of critical importance which need to be firmly established and whose results need to be carefully verified. To keep the process going, the Investigation Committee for the Kyoto Classification of Endoscopic Gastritis and Gastric Cancer Risk was founded. Subsequently, it was decided to develop a universal gastritis classification data entry system and grading system for gastric cancer risk classification that would be suitable for international use based on the Committee's work at the 85th Congress.

As a result of this investigation, the following points were established as guidelines for the entry of endoscopic findings of gastritis:

① Distinguish between *H. pylori*-infected gastritis (currently Infected, active gastritis), *H. pylori*-previously infected gastritis, and *H. pylori*-uninfected gastritis (gastritis absent) and enter them in English (e.g., active gastritis, inactive gastritis, and non-gastritis) so that the system can be used and understood worldwide.

② Enter the extent of atrophy (using Kimura-Takemoto Classification) in parentheses.

③ Enter any other relevant findings in addition to those findings used in the diagnosis of gastritis in ① at the end of the entry after "with".

To achieve this goal, the classifications of *H. pylori* infection conditions and gastritis findings were studied (Table 1 on page 26). The clinical cases (**Cases 1–5**) described below are based on this table and the specified data entry methods for endoscopic findings, but the system may need to be revised as necessary depending on the results of future research. For the grading method for endoscopic findings related to gastric cancer risk, please see Table 1 in Chapter 3-1 on page 102.

2 Entering endoscopic findings of gastritis according to clinical cases

Case 1

Final diagnosis Active gastritis （O-2） A_2 IM_0 H_0 N_0 $DR_{2\ (4)}$

[Description] Atrophy is present with a degree of O-2. Diffuse redness (severe), which is an important finding of infection, can be seen in the corpus. This case should be entered as "active gastritis (O-2)". It is an *H. pylori*-infected case.

[Endoscopic finding grades for gastric cancer risk] Enter A_2 IM_0 H_0 N_0 $DR_{2\ (4)}$ based on the following findings: O-2 atrophy, intestinal metaplasia absent, fold enlargement (hypertrophy) absent, nodularity absent, and diffuse redness present.

Case 2

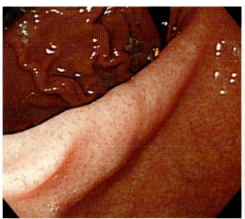
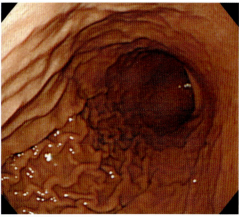

Final diagnosis Non-gastritis with patchy redness of antrum   A0 IM0 H0 N0 DR0 (0)

[Description] Signs of RAC can be seen from the lesser curvature of the angulus to the lesser curvature of the antrum (gastric gland polyp is recognized in the corpus although it is not clear from the pictures). There are no signs of atrophy, intestinal metaplasia, or sticky mucus. Patchy redness can be seen in the pyloric antrum. This case should be entered as "non-gastritis with patchy redness of antrum". It is an *H. pylori*-uninfected case, and the patient was treated with aspirin.

[Endoscopic finding grades for gastric cancer risk] Enter A0 IM0 H0 N0 DR0 (0) based on the following findings: atrophy absent, intestinal metaplasia absent, fold enlargement (hypertrophy) absent, nodularity absent, and diffuse redness absent.

Case 3

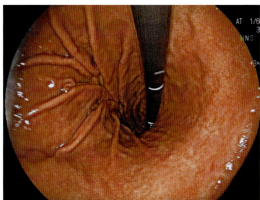
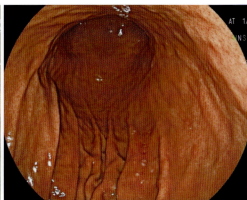

Final diagnosis Inactive-gastritis (C-2)   A1 IM0 H0 N0 DR0 (1)

[Description] Atrophy is present with a degree of C-2. However, there are no findings of *H. pylori* infection, such as sticky mucus, edema, diffuse redness, fold enlargement (hypertrophy), and tortuosity. The border of the atrophic region in the lesser curvature of the corpus is indistinct, and there are partial signs of RAC sign. This case should be entered as "inactive gastritis (C-2)". It is an *H. pylori* previously infected case (3 years after eradication).

[Endoscopic finding grades for gastric cancer risk] Enter A1 IM0 H0 N0 DR0 (1) based on the following findings: C-2 atrophy, intestinal metaplasia absent, fold enlargement (hypertrophy) absent, nodularity absent, and diffuse redness absent.

Case 4

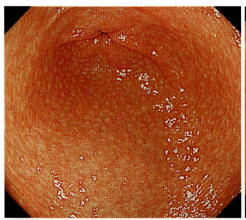
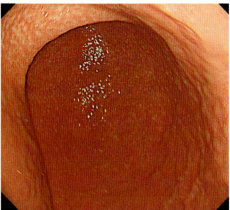
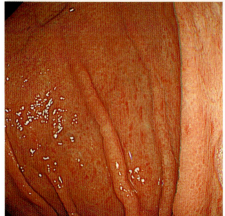

Final diagnosis Active gastritis(C-2) A_1 IM_0 H_0 N_1 $DR_{2\,(4)}$

[Description] Nodularity can be seen in the antrum, and atrophy is present in the lesser curvature of the corpus. The degree of atrophy is C-2. In the greater curvature, diffuse redness and spotty redness can be seen. The patient's age is early 30s. It is an *H. pylori*-infected case. This case should be entered as "active gastritis (C-2)".
[Endoscopic finding grades for gastric cancer risk] Enter A_1 IM_0 H_0 N_1 $DR_{2\,(4)}$ based on the following findings: C-2 atrophy, intestinal metaplasia absent, fold enlargement (hypertrophy) absent, nodularity present, and diffuse redness present.

In the five clinical cases above, the characteristic findings of *H. pylori* infection (current) are diffuse redness, mucosal swelling, fold enlargement (hypertrophy), and sticky mucus. While some of the findings of a past *H. pylori* infection — such as atrophy, xanthoma, and intestinal metaplasia — are also found in current infections, the reverse is not true. Findings characteristic of current infections are not found in past infections, but map-like redness and indistinct atrophic region borders are. Cases in which there is no infection are distinguished by signs of RAC before and after the lesser curvature of the angulus, while findings characteristic of both current and past infections are not found. Classifying gastritis findings according to *H. pylori* infection conditions in this manner makes it possible to diagnose *H. pylori* infection conditions and gastric cancer risks using endoscopic findings.

Case 5

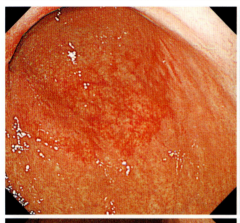
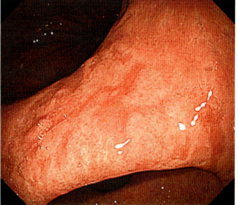

Final diagnosis Inactive-gastritis (C-2)
$A_1\ IM_1\ H_0\ N_0\ DR_{1\ (3)}$

[Description] While diffuse redness and mucosal swelling are not detected in the corpus, atrophy can be seen in the lesser curvature. The degree of atrophy is C-2, but the border of the atrophic region is not clear. Map-like redness can be seen around the antrum and the lesser curvature of the corpus. This case was a follow-up examination of *H. pylori* eradication 10 years before. This case should be entered as "inactive gastritis (C-2)".

[Endoscopic finding grades for gastric cancer risk] Enter $A_1\ IM_1\ H_0\ N_0\ DR_{1\ (3)}$ based on the following findings: C-2 atrophy, intestinal metaplasia present, fold enlargement (hypertrophy) absent, nodularity absent, and diffuse redness absent. Note that RAC had not completely recovered at the time of this examination.

References

1) Dixon MF, Genta RM, Yardley JH, et al : Classification and grading of gastritis. The updated Sydney system. Am J Surg Pathol 1996 ; 20 : 1161-1181
2) Kato T, Yagi N, Kamada T, et al : Diagnosis of *Helicobacter pylori* infection in gastric mucosa by endoscopic features : a multicenter prospective study. Dig Endosc 2013 ; 25 : 508-518
3) Kato M, Terao S, Adachi K, et al : Changes in endoscopic findings of gastritis after cure of *H. pylori* infection : multicenter prospective trial. Dig Endosc 2013 ; 25 : 264-273

Chapter 4 Recording Endoscopic Findings of Gastritis

2. Check Sheet for Background Gastric Mucosa in Endoscopy
—Also usable for checkups for gastric cancer and other gastrointestinal diseases

Kazuhiko Inoue　Tomoari Kamada
Kazunari Murakami　Ken Haruma

The significance of *H. pylori* infection in the development of upper gastrointestinal diseases such as gastric cancer and peptic ulcers makes it critical that its presence or absence be checked not only in everyday gastroenterology practice, but also in examinations for gastric cancer and other gastrointestinal diseases.

Health insurance coverage for *H. pylori* diagnosis and treatment in Japan was expanded in 2013. However, because this expansion of coverage assumes gastritis diagnosis using upper gastrointestinal endoscopy, endoscopy has become more important than ever. As Japan is evolving into what could be called a "super-aging" society, the number of people taking antiplatelet agents such as non-steroidal anti-inflammatory drugs (NSAIDs) and low-dose aspirin (LDA) on a regular basis is increasing rapidly. Similarly, the number of people taking proton pump inhibitors (PPIs) continuously over a long period to treat gastroesophageal reflux disease (GERD) is also increasing. Studying the impact of these drugs on the gastric mucosa is critical.

It should not be difficult for gastrointestinal endoscopy specialists to distinguish between cases not infected with *H. pylori* infection and those suffering continuous infection. They should also have no difficulty assessing endoscopic images after successful *H. pylori* eradication. However, the fact is that the doctors who are actually engaged in primary care and who perform gastric cancer checkups as well as those who use endoscopes in hospitalized overall checkups are not necessarily specialists in gastrointestinal endoscopy.

Now, we have created a check sheet (below) for background gastric mucosa designed to support doctors who are not specialists in endoscopy, enabling them to more easily apprehend the conditions — mainly whether or not there is *H. pylori* infection — of background gastric mucosa.

In this check sheet, the presence/absence and degrees of atrophy are in principle entered according to the Kimura-Takemoto Classification[1]. This will support diagnosis of *H. pylori* infection by encouraging physicians to check for regular arrangement of collecting venules (RAC)[2], fundic gland polyp, red streak, and raised erosion, which are frequently seen among patients not infected *H. pylori* patients, as well as to confirm the presence/absence of diffuse redness, depressive erosion, enlarged fold[3], nodularity[4], and intestinal metaplasia, which are frequently seen among *H. pylori* infected patients. We have also included map-like redness in the gastric mucosa as a referential finding to look for after successful *H. pylori* eradication, while multiple white, flat elevated lesions are listed as an item to be checked for as an effect of PPI medication. If most of the fields in the leftmost column are checked, it is highly likely that the patient is not infected with *H. pylori* and has normal gastric mucosa unaffected by medications.

We are confident that by checking these items, doctors — even those not specialized in gastrointestinal endoscopy — will be able to easily evaluate the presence or absence or *H. pylori* infection.

Check Sheet for Background Gastric Mucosa in Endoscopy

Date of endoscopy:

Name: ID: Sex: Age

Endoscopic diagnosis:

H. pylori infection diagnosis: Uninfected / Infected / After eradiation / Other (   )/ Unknown

Performing doctor:

Endoscopic finding			
RAC	0. Present	1. Absent	
Fundic gland polyp	0. Present	1. Absent	
Red streak	0. Present	1. Absent	
Raised erosion	0. Present	1. Absent	
Atrophy (Kimura-Takemoto Classification)	0. C–0 • C–1	1. C–2 • C–3	2. O–1 or more
Intestinal metaplasia	0. Absent	1. Present	
Enlarged fold	0. Absent	1. Present	
Nodularity	0. Absent	1. Present	
Depressive erosion	0. Absent	1. Present	
Diffuse redness	0. Absent	1. Present	
Map-like redness	0. Absent	1. Present	
Multiple flat and white elevated lesions	0. Absent	1. Present	

References

1) Kimura K and Takemoto T : An endoscopic recognition of the atrophic border and its significance in chronic gastritis. Endoscopy 1969 ; 3 : 87-97
2) Yagi K, Nakamura A and Sekine A : Charactcristic endoscopic and magnified endoscopic findings in the normal stomach without *Helicobacter pylori* infection. J Gastroenterol Hepatol 2002 ; 17 : 39-45
3) Nishibayashi H, Kanayama S, Kiyohara T, et al : *Helicobacter pylori*-induced enlarged-fold gastritis is associated with increased mutagenicity of gastric juice, increased oxidative DNA damage, and an increased risk of gastric carcinoma. J Gastroenterol Hepatol 2003 ; 18 : 1384-1391
4) Kamada T, Hata J, Tanaka A, et al : Nodular gastritis and gastric cancer. Dig Endosc 2006 ; 18 : 79-83

Chapter 4　Recording Endoscopic Findings of Gastritis

3. Endoscopic Diagnosis and Classification of Chronic Gastritis That Conforms to Histological Diagnosis

Shigemi Nakajima　Ryoji Kushima

 Diagnosis policy of chronic gastritis

The diagnosis and classification of histological chronic gastritis are closely connected to the risk of gastric cancer. In other words, the endoscopic diagnosis should not disagree with the histopathological diagnosis. It is also important that endoscopists not only be able to diagnose the presence of chronic gastritis, but also its absence. Currently, histopathological diagnosis should conform to the Updated Sydney System (USS)[1]. Methods for diagnosis and classification of chronic gastritis are proposed below.

Diagnosis of presence/absence and activity of chronic gastritis

Diagnosis of presence/absence and activity of chronic gastritis corresponds with current, previous, and non-infection of *H. pylori* and is classified as follows.

1) Chronic active gastritis (CAG)：current *H. pylori* infection are suspected (Fig. 1)

Neutrophil infiltration, as well as mononuclear cell infiltration, are usually seen in an *H. pylori*-infected stomach. Mononuclear cell infiltration is a finding of chronic gastritis

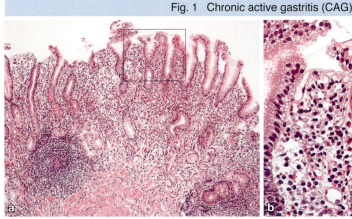

Fig. 1　Chronic active gastritis (CAG)

Magnified image

Atrophic fundic gland mucosa that exhibits lymphoid/plasma cell infiltration and neutrophil infiltration (**b** is a magnified image in the box in **a**)

Fig. 2 Chronic inactive gastritis (CIG)

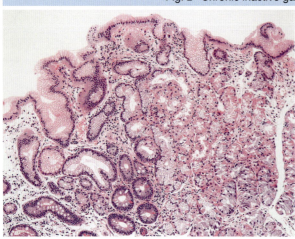

Fundic gland mucosa that exhibits intestinal metaplasia. Although there is minor lymphoid/plasma cell infiltration, neutrophil infiltration is not observed.

while neutrophil infiltration is a finding of acute gastritis. Together, they are called chronic active gastritis (CAG)[1]. If CAG is recognized, there is virtually no doubt that *H. pylori* infection is present. Hence, when current infection of *H. pylori* is suspected endoscopically, it should be diagnosed as CAG.

2) Chronic inactive gastritis (CIG) : *H. pylori* past infection are suspected (Fig. 2)

After *H. pylori* eradication, neutrophil infiltration disappears and the disease becomes inactive. Although there is less mononuclear cell infiltration, the stomach does not return to normal immediately and inflammatory cell infiltration often remains. Pathologically, the condition of gastric mucosa after *H. pylori* eradication is chronic inactive gastritis (CIG).

In addition, there are cases in which past inflammation and mucosal damage are suggested because intestinal metaplasia and atrophy/fibrosis are recognized pathologically although there is virtually no inflammatory cell infiltration. We think that this should be included in CIG because the inflammation sometimes comes to an end in *H. pylori*-past-infected cases while these findings remain. Hence, when past infection of *H. pylori* is suspected endoscopically, it should be diagnosed as CIG.

3) Normal stomach (N) or non-gastritis (NG) (Fig. 3)

When it is determined that a stomach is not infected with *H. pylori* — that is, there is no inflammatory cell infiltration and no CIG finding — it is classified as a histologically normal stomach. However, since pathological diagnosis of atrophy differs depending on the site where the tissue was obtained, the endoscopist must let the pathologist know exactly where the tissue was obtained from[2]. Pathologically, if there is no finding of CIG at all even after *H. pylori* eradication, then the stomach must be diagnosed as normal.

Even in a stomach which has previously been infected with *H. pylori*, similar endoscopic findings to those of a normal stomach may be exhibited. Such a stomach is probably close enough to a pathologically normal stomach to be diagnosed as endoscopically normal as well. In such a case, "normal stomach" does not necessarily mean "not infected with *H. pylori*"; rather, it would mean that the gastric mucosa is *H. pylori*-uninfected or equivalent. Gastric mucosa equivalent to a normal stomach not infected

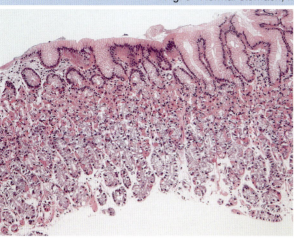

Fig. 3 Normal stomach, non-gastritis

Gastric fundic gland mucosa with virtually no inflammatory cell infiltration.

with *H. pylori* can be endoscopically classified as normal (N) or non-gastritis (NG).

3 Diagnosis of atrophy

Atrophy of the gastric mucosa is strongly related to the risk of gastric cancer. Thus, when diagnosing the background gastric mucosa, it is advisable to diagnose the presence/absence and degree of atrophy at the same time. For the diagnosis of atrophy, Kimura-Takemoto Classification[2)-5)] should be used (Fig. 2 on page 11). In the future, this classification will need to be made more consistent with histological diagnosis of atrophy. It will also have to be simplified so that it can be used worldwide to support diagnosis of gastric cancer risk.

4 Consistency with pathological diagnosis

To the extent possible, the pathologist should perform pathological diagnosis in accordance with the visual analogue scale (see Fig. 3 in reference 1) in the USS[1)]. Keep in mind that it has been reported that it is difficult to reproduce the assessment of atrophy. To ensure consistency with the endoscopic diagnosis, it is advisable to ask the pathologist to indicate, at least, the degree of neutrophil infiltration and the presence/absence of intestinal metaplasia.

References

1) Dixon MF, Genta RM, Yardley JH, et al : Classification and grading of gastritis. The Updated Sydney System. Am J Surg Pathol 1996 ; 20 : 1161-1181
2) Nakajima S, Sakaki N, Hattori T : [Topography of histological gastritis and endoscopic findings.] Helicobacter Research 2009; 13: 74-81 (In Japanese)
3) Kimura K : Chronological transition of the fundic-pyloric border determined by stepwise biopsy of the lesser and greater curvatures of the stomach. Gastroenterology 1972 ; 63 : 584-592
4) Kimura K and Takemoto T : An endoscopic recognition of the atrophic border and its significance in chronic gastritis. Endoscopy 1969 ; 1(3) : 87-97

5) Sakaki N, Okazaki Y, Takemoto T. [Gland boundaries and endoscopy. Takemoto T, Kawai K ed: Topics of gastrointestinal endoscopy.] Tokyo: Igaku Tosho Shuppan. 1978: 178–183. (In Japanese.)

Index

A

abdominal pain 72, 73, 74
active gastritis 114, 116
acute gastric mucosal lesion (AGML) 9
AFI (Autofluorescence Imaging) 28
antithrombotic agent 29, 78
antrum-predominant gastritis 67, 100
areae gastricae 48
aspirin 77, 78, 85, 87, 118
atrophic gastritis 27, 30, 83, 99
atrophy 30, 31, 32, 59, 89, 101, 114, 115, 116, 118, 119, 122
autoimmune gastritis 17, 113

B

BLI (Blue Laser Imaging) 92, 93, 102

C

Classification of the Study Group for Establishing Endoscopic Diagnosis of Chronic Gastritis 14
check sheet for background gastric mucosa in endoscopy 118, 119
closed type 32
chronic active gastritis (CAG) 26, 121
chronic inactive gastritis (CIG) 28, 122
cobblestone mucosa 94
corpus erosion 79, 80, 81, 82
corpus linear erosion 80, 82
corpus-predominant gastritis 100
crest erosion 79, 82
currently *H. pylori*-infected gastric mucosa 26, 114
cytomegalovirus (CMV) 65

D

depressive erosion 63, 64, 65, 118, 119
diffuse redness 16, 38, 39, 40, 41, 42, 43, 45, 90, 102, 104, 106, 107, 108, 109, 110, 114, 116, 118, 119
disappearance/reduction of —— 42
dilated cystic gland 70

E

edematous mucosa 44
endoscopic atrophic border 14
enlarged folds 44, 102, 104, 108, 109, 110, 118, 119
——, tortuous folds 49, 50
—— gastritis 28
epithelial cell deficiency 65
erosion 63, 64, 65, 72, 79, 80, 81, 82, 85, 86, 118
erosive gastritis 16

F

familial adenomatous polyposis (FAP) 70
FICE (Flexible spectral Imaging Color Enhancement) 93
flat erosion 82
foveolar-hyperplastic polyp 25, 57–59
functional dyspepsia (FD) 9
fundic gland polyp 68, 69, 70, 118, 119
fundic gland region 70

G

gastric adenoma 37
gastric cancer in young patients 56
gastric mucosal bleeding 78
giant fold, giant ruga 51
grading endoscopic findings

related to gastric cancer risk 102
grayish white elevation 34
grayish white mucosa 34, 37

H

H_2 receptor antagonist 93
HE-staining 54, 91
Helicobacter pylori (*H. pylori*) 9, 15, 25
——-infected gastritis 25, 113
——-uninfected gastric mucosa 25, 114, 122
previously —— -infected gastric mucosa 28, 114
types of gastritis associated with —— -infecttion 100
hematin 72, 77, 78, 80, 86
Hirafuku's Classification 17
histological gastritis 9
histopathological classification of gastritis 16
histopathological diagnosis 121
history of the classification of gastritis 11

I

image enhanced endoscopy (IEE) 37, 101, 102
inactive gastritis 114, 115, 117
indigo carmine spraying 52, 53, 57, 60, 80, 84, 91, 92
inflammatory cell infiltration 31, 47, 99, 122
intestinal metaplasia 33–37, 89–99, 107–108, 110, 118–119, 122, 124
iron-deficiency anemia 25, 59

K

Kimura-Takemoto Classification 10, 11, 14, 27,

32, 104, 118, 123

Kyoto Classification of Gastritis 11, 26, 113

L

light blue crest (LBC)   28, 35, 37, 102, 110

lymphoid follicle 56, 101

M

malignant lymphoma 28

map-like redness   87, 88, 89, 90, 117, 118, 119

metaplastic gastritis 28

methylene blue dye 102

mononuclear cell infiltration 28, 42

morphological gastritis 9

mucosa associated lymphoid tissue (MALT) lymphoma 25

mucosal swelling   3, 46, 47, 48

multiple white and flat elevated lesion 91, 92, 93, 118, 119

N

NBI (Narrow Band Imaging) 28, 35, 37, 60, 61, 63, 68, 69, 83, 85, 91, 93, 102, 110

neutrophil infiltration   25, 42, 121, 124

nodularity   52, 53, 54, 55, 56, 102, 106, 118, 119

nodular gastritis 11, 28, 54, 56, 101

nodules 56

non-gastritis 114, 115

normal gastric mucosa 70

normal stomach 25, 122

NSAID 64, 78, 86, 87, 118

O

"octopus-sucker" erosion (verrucous gastritis) 76, 82

OLGA Staging 100

OLGIM Staging 100

open type 32

P

pangastritis 100

patchy redness   17, 83, 84, 85, 86, 90, 115

peptic ulcer 9, 25

pink speckling 74

plasma cell infiltration 122, 123

portal hypertension gastric disease 44, 45

previously *H. pylori*-infected gastric mucosa 28, 114

proton pump inhibitor (PPI) 18, 29, 37, 70, 80, 93, 118

pseudopyloric gland metaplasia 99

punctiform 16

R

raised erosion   16, 75, 76, 79, 80, 82, 118, 119

recording endoscopic findings of gastritis 113

red streak   71, 72, 73, 74, 75, 81, 118, 119

reflux esophagitis 91, 93

regular arrangement of collecting venules (RAC) 16, 25, 66, 67, 71, 115, 118, 119

risk of gastric cancer 99, 113

round vacuolated cells 62

S

Sakita's Classification 13

Schindler's Classification   10, 12, 113

Strickland & Mackay classification of chronic gastritis 17

Structure Enhancement 42, 45

spotty redness   43, 44, 45, 90, 116

Sydney System 11, 15

symptomatic gastritis 9

T

Tasaka's Classification 13

Type A gastritis 17, 32, 99

Type B gastritis 17

types of gastritis associated with *H. pylori* infection 100

U

Updated Sydney System (USS) 11, 76, 113, 121

undifferentiated gastric cancer 28, 56, 99

V

vascular pattern 32

varioliform 16

W

white coating 59

Whitehead's Classification 16

white opaque substance (WOS) 35, 37, 102

X

xanthoma 60, 61, 62

Y

Yamada's Type II polyp 57, 68

Yamagata's Classification 13